Small Animal ECGs

Dedication

*To my family: my wife Mary
and our three sons, David, Dennis and Sean*

Small Animal ECGs
An introductory guide
Third Edition

Mike Martin

WILEY Blackwell

This edition first published 2015 © 2015 by John Wiley & Sons, Ltd

Second edition published 2007 © by Mike Martin
First edition published 2000 © by Mike Martin

Registered office:
John Wiley & Sons, Ltd, The Atrium, Southern Gate, Chichester, West Sussex, PO19 8SQ, UK

Editorial offices:
9600 Garsington Road, Oxford, OX4 2DQ, UK
The Atrium, Southern Gate, Chichester, West Sussex, PO19 8SQ, UK
1606 Golden Aspen Drive, Suites 103 and 104, Ames, Iowa 50010, USA

For details of our global editorial offices, for customer services and for information about how to apply for permission to reuse the copyright material in this book please see our website at www.wiley.com/wiley-blackwell

Library of Congress Cataloging-in-Publication Data

Martin, Mike W. S., author.
  Small animal ECGs : an introductory guide / Mike Martin. – Third edition.
    p. ; cm.
  Includes bibliographical references and index.
  Summary: "Small Animal ECGs: An Introductory Guide provides all the information that veterinarians need when using electrocardiography techniques for the first time" – Provided by publisher.
  ISBN 978-1-118-40973-2 (paperback)
1. Veterinary electrocardiography. I. Title. II. Title: Small animal electrocardiography.
  [DNLM: 1. Electrocardiography–veterinary. 2. Animals, Domestic. SF 811]

SF811.M37 2015
636.089′61207547 – dc23

                    2015007744

A catalogue record for this book is available from the British Library.

Wiley also publishes its books in a variety of electronic formats. Some content that appears in print may not be available in electronic books.

Typeset in 9.5/11.5pt MinionPro by SPi Global, Chennai, India
Printed and bound by CPI Group (UK) Ltd, Croydon CR0 4YY

C9781118409732_211223

Contents

Preface to third edition

Yet again, this new edition comes with a significant amount of change and update, but the target audience remains the beginners, from veterinary graduates and students to nurses and technicians. It remains an easy-to-read introduction to ECGs. Usefully, it also includes an explanation of the clinical findings with each arrhythmia, what the rhythm might sound like on auscultation and when there is a pulse deficit.

For this edition I also asked a number of friends and colleagues in the world of cardiology for suggestions, tips and advice. These have been incorporated into this edition, so please also read the acknowledgements.

So I hear you ask, What are the changes? The general flow of the book remains unchanged, but some chapters have been divided to further improve explanation and understanding. There are extra chapters on Holter monitoring, with one explaining the mechanisms of supraventricular tachycardias (which is a new development to our knowledge and the available treatment – ablation). There are additional sections explaining compensatory pauses, fusion complexes and Ashman's phenomenon. There is a larger section on accelerated idioventricular rhythm (AIVR), which has been an increasingly recognised arrhythmia.

Finally, the book is now in colour, which I hope provides a more enjoyable read. All the ECG tracings are new and reproduced in colour. The line diagrams are now all beautifully illustrated in colour, which adds to easier understanding and explanation.

The continuing positive feedback and demand for a third edition has been great. Thanks!

Mike Martin

About the author

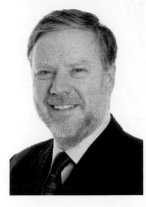

Mike Martin graduated from University College Dublin in 1986. He worked for 2 years in mixed practice and 4 years at the Royal (Dick) School of Veterinary Studies, University of Edinburgh, as a House-Physician and then as Resident in Veterinary Cardiology. During this time, he gained the Royal College of Veterinary Surgeons (RCVS) Certificate and Diploma in Veterinary Cardiology and then RCVS Specialist status in Veterinary Cardiology in 1995, which has been re-validated every 5 years ever since. He has since been an examiner for the RCVS at Certificate and Diploma level.

He has been working at his own, private, referral practice since 1992 (over 20 years) and has published over 40 scientific peer-reviewed papers. He is a frequent CPD lecturer within Europe and has presented his clinical research at Specialist Cardiology meetings in both Europe and the United States. He has been both Honorary Secretary and Chairman of the Veterinary Cardiovascular Society. He is author of two textbooks: Small Animal ECGs: An Introductory Guide (3rd edition) and Cardiorespiratory Diseases of the Dog and Cat (2nd edition) published by Wiley and has written a number of book chapters in Veterinary Textbooks.

He is a recipient of BSAVA awards: in 1993, the Dunkin Award; in 2000, the Melton Award; in 2006, the PetSavers Award; and in 2010, the Dunkin and Blaine Awards.

Acknowledgements

I would like to thank all those who have assisted in the production of this book, from those in the audience during lectures who provided feedback to my colleagues, peers and friends.

More importantly, after being asked by Wiley to produce a third edition of this book, I sought opinions from a number of friends and colleagues in the world of veterinary cardiology. Their suggestions, tips and advice have been very helpful such that I hope this edition of the book has further evolved and progressed to be an even better and more useful book. Additionally, I aimed to replace all the ECG tracings in the book to give it a fresh look, and this also needed a call for help from my colleagues to obtain good quality examples of these. The photographs which have been provided by colleagues are acknowledged in the figure legends.

So a very appreciative thanks goes to:

Dr. Paul Wotton, formerly RCVS Specialist in Veterinary Cardiology
Honorary Senior Veterinary Clinician in Cardiology, University of Glasgow

Jo Duke McEwan, RCVS Specialist in Veterinary Cardiology
Senior Lecturer in Small Animal Cardiology, University of Liverpool

Geoff Culshaw, RCVS Specialist in Veterinary Cardiology
Senior Lecturer in Cardiopulmonary Medicine, University of Edinburgh

Anne French, RCVS Specialist in Veterinary Cardiology
Senior Veterinary Clinician in Cardiology, University of Glasgow

Simon Dennis, RCVS Specialist in Veterinary Cardiology
Lecturer in Veterinary Cardiology, University of Pennsylvania

Nicole Van Israel, European Specialist in Veterinary Cardiology
Animal Cardiopulmonary Consultancy, Masta, Belgium

Yolanda Martinez Pereira, RCVS Specialist in Veterinary Cardiology
Lecturer in Veterinary Cardiology, University of Edinburgh

Stephen Collins, RCVS Specialist in Veterinary Cardiology
Southern Counties Veterinary Specialists, Ringwood, England

Jo Harris, CertVC
Resident in Veterinary Cardiology, HeartVets

Dave Dickson, CertVC
Resident in Veterinary Cardiology, HeartVets

Abbreviations

+ve	positive (electrode)
−ve	negative (electrode)
AF	Atrial fibrillation
AIVR	Accelerated idioventricular rhythm
APC	Atrial premature complex
ARVC	Arrhythmogenic right ventricular cardiomyopathy
AV	Atrioventricular
AVN	Atrioventricular node
CKCS	Cavalier King Charles spaniel (dog)
DSH	Domestic short hair (cat)
ECG	Electrocardiogram
FAT	focal atrial tachycardia
GSD	German Shepherd dog
HCM	Hypertrophic cardiomyopathy
i/v	intravenous (injection)
JPC	Junctional premature complex
LA	left atrium
LAFB	left anterior fascicular block
LBBB	left bundle branch block
LF	left fore (leg)
LH	left hind (leg)
LV	left ventricle
LVE	left ventricular enlargement
MEA	mean electrical axis
MVD	Mitral valve disease
OAVRT	orthodromic atrioventricular reciprocating tachycardia
PDA	patent ductus arteriosus
RA	right atrium
RBBB	right bundle branch block
RF	right fore (leg)
RH	right hind (leg)
RV	right ventricle
RVE	right ventricular enlargement
SA	Sinoatrial
SAN	Sinoatrial node
SVPC	Supraventricular premature complex
SVT	Supraventricular tachycardia
TIMF	Tachycardia-induced myocardial failure
VPC	Ventricular premature complex
VF	Ventricular fibrillation
VT	Ventricular tachycardia
WHWT	West Highland White terrier (dog)

PART 1
Understanding the electricity of the heart and how it produces an ECG complex

1 • What is an ECG?

An **electrocardiograph** (ECG), in its simplest form, is a voltmeter (or galvanometer) that records the changing electrical activity in the heart by means of positive (+ve) and negative (−ve) electrodes (Fig. 1.1). **Electrocardiography** is the process of recording these changing potential differences.

A +ve and a −ve electrode can be placed almost anywhere on, or in, the body to record electrical changes. One of the most common and simplest methods is to place these electrodes on the limbs of animals – referred to as a **body surface limb ECG recording.** However, if monitoring an ECG during anaesthesia or echocardiography, for example, it is sufficient to place the −ve electrode anywhere cranial to the heart (e.g. the forelimb or neck) and the +ve electrode caudal to the heart (e.g. the hind limb, abdomen or flank). Electrodes can also be placed on the chest (precordial chest ECG recording – commonly used in humans) or inside the cardiac chambers (used in electrophysiological studies). This book focuses on the conventional limb ECG recording, which is the method most commonly used in veterinary medicine for clinical diagnosis of arrhythmias.

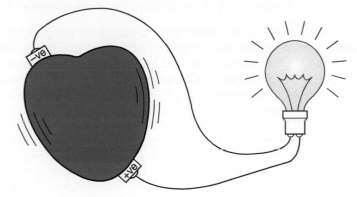

Figure 1.1 An ECG records the 'electricity of the heart'.

Small Animal ECGs: An Introductory Guide, Third Edition. Mike Martin.
© 2015 John Wiley & Sons, Ltd. Published 2015 by John Wiley & Sons, Ltd.

2 • The electricity of the heart

Electrical coordination of atrioventricular contraction

For the heart to function efficiently as a 'circulatory pump', it must have a coordinated contraction: the two atria contracting and passing blood into the two ventricles, followed by contraction of the ventricles, pumping blood into the aorta and pulmonary artery; that is, there must be a coordinated atrioventricular (AV) contraction. In order for the cardiac muscle cells to contract, they must first receive an electrical stimulus. It is this electrical activity that is detected by an ECG.

The electrical stimulus must first depolarise the two atria. Then, after an appropriate time interval, it must depolarise the two ventricles. The heart must then repolarise (and 'refill') in time for the next stimulus and contraction. Additionally, it must repeatedly do so, increasing in rate with an increase in demand and conversely slowing at rest.

Formation of the normal P–QRS–T complex

All cells within the heart have the potential to generate their own electrical activity; however, the **sinoatrial** (SA) **node** is the fastest part of the electrical circuit to do so and is therefore the 'rate controller', termed the **pacemaker**. The sinus node rate is, therefore, the dominant pacemaker (over the other cells in the heart) by being the fastest and by a mechanism termed **overdrive suppression**. The rate of the SA node is influenced by the balance in the autonomic tone, that is, the sympathetic (increases rate) and parasympathetic (decreases rate) systems.

The electrical discharge for each cardiac cycle (Fig. 2.1) starts in the SA node. Depolarisation spreads through the atrial muscle cells. The

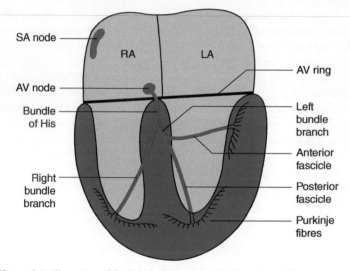

Figure 2.1 Illustration of the heart's electrical circuit. SA – sinoatrial; AV – atrioventricular; RA – right atrium; LA – left atrium.

depolarisation wave then spreads through the **AV node;** however, it does so at a relatively slower rate, creating a delay. Conduction passes through the AV ring (from the atria into the ventricles) through a narrow pathway called the **bundle of His.** This then divides in the ventricular septum into **left and right bundle branches** (going to the left and right ventricles). The left bundle branch divides further into **anterior and posterior fascicles.** The conduction tissue spreads into the myocardium as very fine branches called **Purkinje fibres.**

Formation of the P wave

The SA node is therefore the start of the electrical depolarisation wave. This depolarisation wave spreads through the atria (somewhat like the ripples in water created by dropping a stone into it). As the parts of the atria nearest to the SA node are depolarised (Fig. 2.2), it creates an electrical **potential difference** between the depolarised atria and the parts that are not yet depolarised (i.e. still in a resting state).

If negative (−ve) and positive (+ve) electrodes were placed approximately in line with those shown in the diagram (Fig. 2.2), then this would result in the voltmeter (i.e. the ECG machine) detecting the depolarisation wave travelling from the SA node, across the atria, in the general direction of the +ve electrode. On the ECG recording, all positive deflections are displayed as an upward (i.e. positive) deflection on the ECG paper, and negative deflections are displayed downwards. The atrial depolarisation wave, therefore, creates an upward excursion of the stylus on the ECG paper.

When the whole of the atria become depolarised, then there is no longer an electrical potential difference, thus, the stylus returns to its idle position – referred to as the **baseline.** The brief upward deflection of the stylus on the ECG paper creates the P wave, representing the atrial electrical activity (Fig. 2.3). The muscle mass of the atria is fairly small, thus, the electrical changes associated with depolarisation are also small.

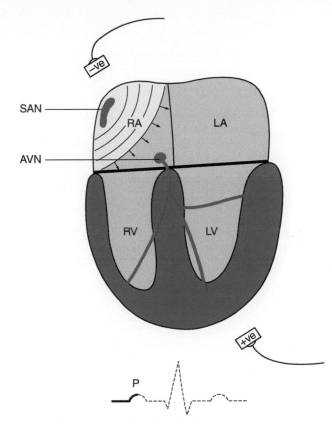

Figure 2.2 Illustration of partial depolarisation of the atria and formation of the P wave. The shaded area represents the depolarised myocardial cells; the arrows represent the direction in which the depolarisation wave travels. RA – right atrium; LA – left atrium; RV – right ventricle; LV – left ventricle; SAN – sinoatrial node; AVN – atrioventricular node.

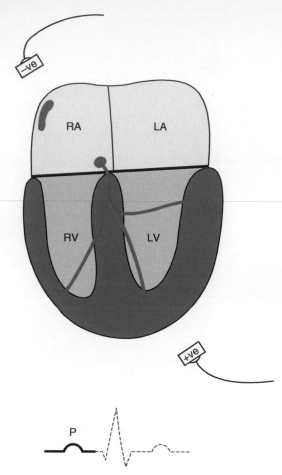

Figure 2.3 Illustration of complete depolarisation of the atria and formation of the P wave. RA – right atrium; LA – left atrium; RV – right ventricle; LV – left ventricle.

The P–R interval

During the course of atrial depolarisation, the depolarisation wave also depolarises the AV node. The speed at which the electrical depolarisation wave travels through the AV node is deliberately slow so that ventricular contraction will be correctly coordinated following atrial contraction. Once the depolarisation wave passes through the AV node, it travels very rapidly through the specialised conduction tissues of the ventricles, that is, the bundle of His, the left and right bundle branches and Purkinje fibres.

The formation of the QRS complex

The Q waves

Initially the first part of the ventricles to depolarise is the ventricular septum, with a small depolarisation wave that travels in a direction away from the +ve electrode (Fig. 2.4). This creates a small downward, or negative, deflection on the ECG paper – termed the Q wave.

The R wave

Subsequently the bulk of the ventricular myocardium is depolarised. This creates a depolarisation wave that travels towards the +ve electrode (Fig. 2.5). As it is a large mass of muscle tissue, it usually creates a large deflection – this is termed the R wave.

The S wave

Following depolarisation of the majority of the ventricles, the only remaining parts are basilar portions. This creates a depolarisation wave that travels away from the +ve electrode and is a small mass of tissue (Fig. 2.6). Thus, this creates a small negative deflection on the ECG paper – the S wave.

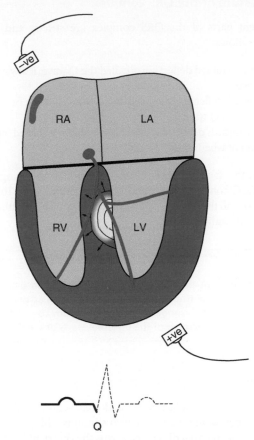

Figure 2.4 Illustration of depolarisation of the ventricular septum and formation of the Q wave. RA – right atrium; LA – left atrium; RV – right ventricle; LV – left ventricle.

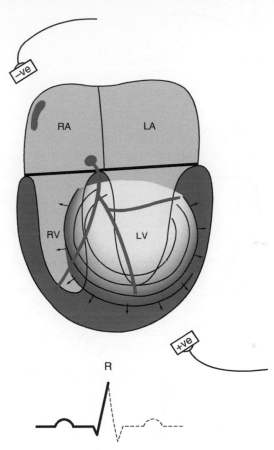

Figure 2.5 Illustration of depolarisation of the bulk of the ventricular myocardium and formation of the R wave. RA – right atrium; LA – left atrium; RV – right ventricle; LV – left ventricle.

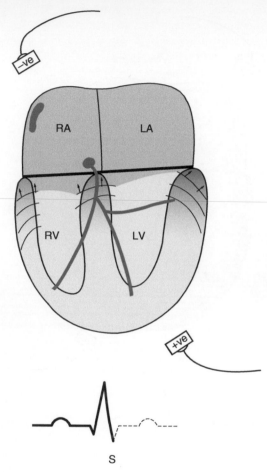

Figure 2.6 Illustration of depolarisation of the basilar portions of the ventricles and formation of the S wave. RA – right atrium; LA – left atrium; RV – right ventricle; LV – left ventricle.

Nomenclature of the QRS complex

The different parts of the QRS complex are strictly and arbitrarily labelled as follows:

- The first downward deflection is called the Q wave; it always precedes the R wave.
- Any upward deflection is called the R wave; it may or may not be preceded by a Q wave.
- Any downward deflection after an R wave is called an S wave, regardless of whether there is a Q wave or not.

However, this fairly rigid terminology becomes confusing when the shapes of ECG complexes vary and become complicated. Therefore, in this book, we will think of the '**QRS complex**' as a whole, rather than try to recognise its individual parts.

> **Note**
>
> While the different parts of the QRS waveform can be identified, it is often easier to think of the 'whole ventricular depolarisation waveform' as the **QRS complex**. This will avoid any confusion over the correct and proper naming of the different parts of the QRS complex.

The T wave

Following complete depolarisation (and contraction) of the ventricles, they then repolarise in time for the next stimulus. This phase of repolarisation creates a potential difference across the ventricular myocardium, until it is completely repolarised. This results in a deflection from the baseline – termed the T wave (Fig. 2.7).

The T wave in dogs and cats is very variable, and it can be negative or positive or even biphasic (i.e. a combination of both). This is because repolarisation of the myocardium in small animals is slightly random, unlike in humans, for example, where repolarisation is very organised and always results in a positive T wave. Thus, the diagnostic value obtainable from the abnormalities in the T wave of small animals is very limited, unlike the useful features of the abnormal T waveforms seen in humans.

The repolarisation wave of the atria (T_a) is rarely recognised on a surface ECG, as it is very small and is usually hidden within the QRS complex.

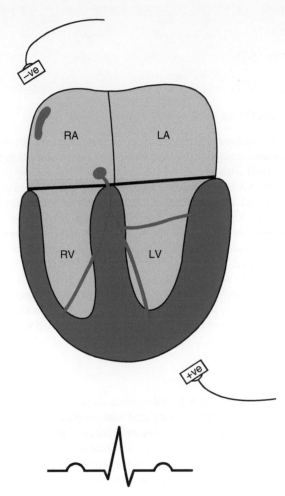

Figure 2.7 Illustration of complete depolarisation and repolarisation of the ventricles and completion of the P–QRS–T complex. RA – right atrium; LA – left atrium; RV – right ventricle; LV – left ventricle.

3 • Rhythms of sinus origin

Rhythms of sinus origin

The formation of the normal ECG complex has been explained in the preceding chapter; this normal complex is termed a **sinus complex.** A sequence of beats originating from the SA node will form a sinus rhythm. Four common sinus rhythms are described as follows.

Sinus rhythm

The stimulus originates from the SA node (dominant pacemaker) regularly at a constant rate, depolarising the atria and ventricles and normally producing a coordinated atrioventricular contraction. This is a normal rhythm.

ECG characteristics

There is a normal P wave followed by a normal QRS complex with a T wave. The rhythm is regular (constant) and the rate is within normal for age and breed (Fig. 3.1).

The size of the ECG complexes are typically small in cats (Fig. 3.2). Obtaining an artefact-free tracing is therefore important (in cats) in order to identify clearly all the parts of the ECG complexes.

Clinical findings

There are regular heart sounds on auscultation (i.e. lubb-dub, lubb-dub, lubb-dub . . . .) with a pulse for each heartbeat and at a rate that is normal for age, breed and species.

Small Animal ECGs: An Introductory Guide, Third Edition. Mike Martin.
© 2015 John Wiley & Sons, Ltd. Published 2015 by John Wiley & Sons, Ltd.

Sinus arrhythmia

The stimulus originates from the SA node, but the rate varies (increases and decreases) regularly. This is a normal and common rhythm in dogs. It is associated with an increase in parasympathetic activity (i.e. vagal tone) on the SA node. There is commonly a regular variation in rate often associated with respiration (i.e. it speeds up and slows down), and it is, therefore, often called **respiratory sinus arrhythmia.** Since sinus arrhythmia is an indicator of increased parasympathetic tone, conversely, it is also an indicator of reduced sympathetic tone. In dogs with heart failure, one of the compensatory responses is an increase in sympathetic tone and therefore, normal sinus arrhythmia is often lost, and a sinus tachycardia develops. Sinus arrhythmia is uncommon in cats, when in-clinic, and it might be seen in association with dyspnoea. However, it can be seen on the Holter recordings obtained while relaxing at home.

ECG characteristics

There is a normal P wave followed by normal QRS–T waves. The rhythm varies in rate; this is often associated with respiration (Fig. 3.3). The rhythm can sometimes be described as being regularly irregular, that is, the variation in rate is fairly regular. The rate is within normal for age and breed. It is also common, with sinus arrhythmia, to see a variation in the P-wave morphology; this is termed a **wandering pacemaker** (Chapter 8).

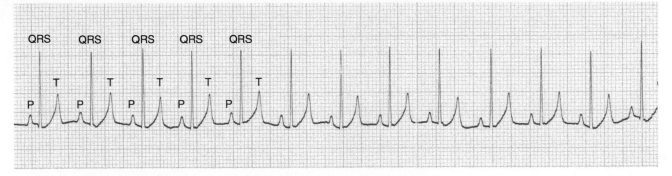

Figure 3.1 ECG from a dog showing a normal sinus rhythm at a rate of 140/min (25 mm/s and 10 mm/mV).

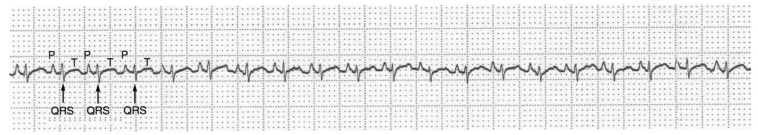

Figure 3.2 ECG from a cat showing a normal sinus rhythm at a rate of 210/min (25 mm/s and 10 mm/mV).

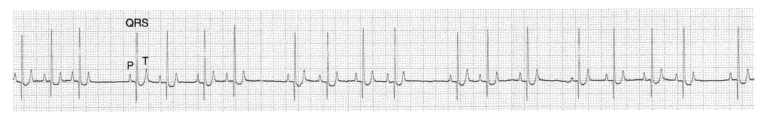

Figure 3.3 ECG from a dog showing a normal respiratory sinus arrhythmia at a rate of 110/min (25 mm/s and 10 mm/mV).

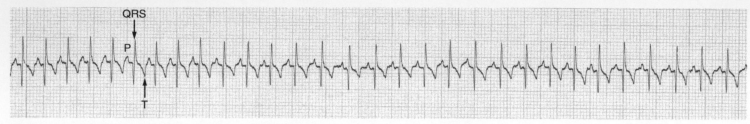

Figure 3.4 ECG from nervous Weimaraner. There is a sinus tachycardia at 210/min (25 mm/s and 5 mm/mV).

Clinical findings

The heart rhythm varies on auscultation with some regularity – increasing and decreasing in rate, with a pulse for every heartbeat and at a rate that is normal for age, breed and species.

Sinus tachycardia

The SA node generates an impulse and depolarisation at a rate that is faster than normal.

ECG characteristics

There is a sinus rhythm but at a faster rate than normal (Fig. 3.4).

Clinical findings

The heart rate is faster than normal for age and breed, with a pulse for every heartbeat (although with faster rates, the pulse may become weaker).

Sinus bradycardia

The SA node generates an impulse and depolarisation at a rate slower than normal. This can be a normal feature in some giant-breed dogs and in athletically fit dogs.

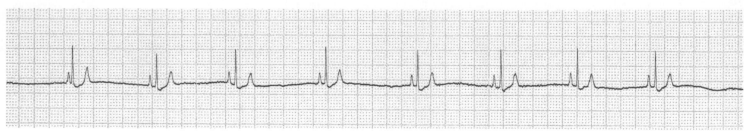

Figure 3.5 ECG from a WHWT dog with a sinus bradycardia at 50/min (25 mm/s and 10 mm/mV).

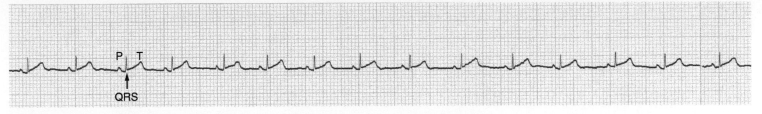

Figure 3.6 ECG from a cat following sedation, showing a sinus bradycardia at 110/min (25 mm/s and 10 mm/mV).

ECG characteristics

There is a sinus rhythm but at a slower rate than normal (Fig. 3.5 and 3.6).

Clinical findings

The heart rate is slower than normal for age and breed, with a pulse for every heartbeat.

PART 2
Abnormal electricity of the heart

4 • Recognising and understanding ectopia

Recognising and understanding ectopia

Arrhythmia and dysrhythmia are synonymous terms, meaning an abnormal rhythm. Arrhythmias include abnormalities in rate, abnormalities associated with ectopia and abnormalities in conduction. Arrhythmias that are essentially slow are referred to as **bradyarrhythmias** (Chapter 7), and those that are fast are referred to as **tachyarrhythmias** (Chapters 4–6).

First identify the morphology of the *normal* QRS complex

Chapter 2 explained the formation of a normal sinus complex. It is important when examining an ECG tracing to identify (from the ECG recording) the normal sinus complex for that animal. Note the shape of the ventricular depolarisation and repolarisation waves, that is, the QRS complex and T wave. To produce shape of QRS and T, depolarisation of the ventricles has occurred by conduction from (or through) the AV node, that is, ventricular depolarisation has been initiated from the AV node (Chapter 2). It is of paramount importance in any tracing, especially if there are a variety of shapes of QRS complexes, to determine which shape represents conduction that has arisen (correctly) via the AV node.

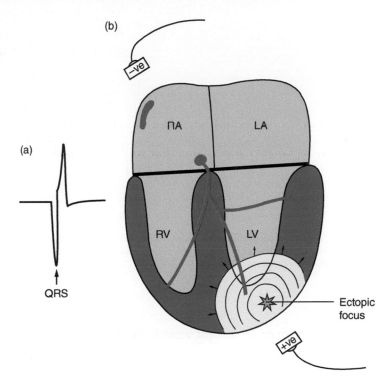

Figure 4.1 Diagram illustrating an ectopic focus with the spreading out of the depolarisation wave (b) and the formation of a QRS–T complex (a) associated with the ventricular ectopic. RA – right atrium; LA – left atrium; RV – right ventricle; LV – left ventricle.

Small Animal ECGs: An Introductory Guide, Third Edition. Mike Martin.
© 2015 John Wiley & Sons, Ltd. Published 2015 by John Wiley & Sons, Ltd.

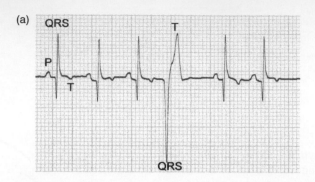

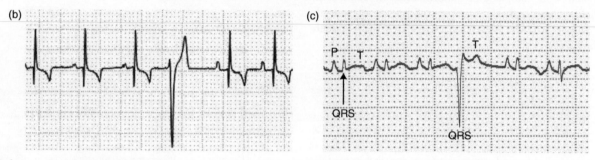

Figure 4.2 ECGs from a collie dog with mitral valve disease (a), a Doberman with preclinical DCM (b) and a DSH cat with HCM (c), each showing a 'typical' ventricular ectopic complex. First, identify the QRS and T morphology for the normal sinus complexes (first three complexes and last two), then the 'wide and bizarre' shaped complex (fourth complex), which must therefore be a ventricular ectopic. (25 mm/s and 10 mm/mV). Fig. 4.2b courtesy of Jo Dukes McEwan.

The morphology of an ectopic *ventricular* depolarisation

Any QRS–T complex, therefore, that is of a **different** shape (compared to the QRS–T of a normal sinus complex *for animal)* represents an abnormality. When the QRS–T complex is different from the normal sinus complex, depolarisation has *(almost certainly)* not arisen via the AV node (which would have produced a normal QRS shape) but from

an ectopic location in the ventricles.[1] Additionally, these ventricular ectopic complexes are not associated with a preceding P wave (except by coincidence).

---

[1] Except when there is aberrant conduction, see Chapter 11. However this is not common.

From Fig. 4.1, it can be seen that the direction of ventricular depolarisation is different from that of the depolarisation arising from the AV node (cf. figures in Chapters 2 and 3). In this example, the ventricular ectopic depolarisation wave is away from the +ve electrode and is, therefore, displayed on the ECG paper as below the baseline, that is, the QRS complex is negative. Secondly, because conduction has not travelled through the normal (therefore, fast) electrical conduction tissue (it has depolarised the ventricular muscle mass from 'cell to cell'), the time it takes to depolarise the ventricles is prolonged. Thus, not only is the QRS complex of the ventricular ectopic different in shape, but it is also prolonged (it takes a longer time). Quite often, the T wave following the QRS complex of a ventricular ectopic is large and opposite in direction to the QRS (Fig 4.2 a, b).

Ventricular ectopic complexes can arise from any part of the ventricles, and thus the direction in which they depolarise the ventricles is variable. In other words, since the direction in which the depolarisation wave travels in relation to the +ve electrode is variable, the shape and magnitude of the QRS complex of a ventricular complex will also be variable (Fig. 4.3).

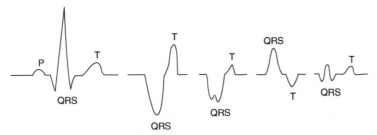

Figure 4.3 Illustration of a normal complex (first complex), followed by four examples of QRS–T complexes with an abnormal morphology due to ventricular ectopic depolarisation. It is paramount to identify the morphology of the QRS complex associated with a sinus complex (first complex). Any QRS complexes of a different morphology (for the animal) must have arisen from an ectopic ventricular focus.

The important point is that the QRS of a ventricular ectopic complex is **different** from the QRS complex that has arisen from the AV node and travelled normally down the electrical conducting tissue to the ventricles (Fig. 4.4).

A ventricular ectopic complex (Fig 4.5) can occur quickly (or early) and is, therefore, termed a **ventricular** *premature* **complex**(VPC)(Figs 4.2 & 4.4). If a ventricular ectopic occurs after a pause (or with delay), then it is referred to as a **ventricular** *escape* **complex** (Fig. 4.6).

On the basis of what has been learned so far, this explanation can also be summarised using a flow chart (Fig 4.7). First, identify the shape of the normal QRS and T complexes for the animal and compare them to those that are different (from normal). These different shaped QRS and T complexes must represent a depolarisation that has not travelled down the AV node; therefore, this must be a ventricular ectopic. Ventricular ectopics can then be classified as premature or escapes.

> **Note**
>
> That the term 'beat' implies that there has been an actual contraction. In 'ECG-speak', it is better to use the term **complex** or **depolarisation** to describe the waveforms on the electrocardiograph.

> **Key points**
>
> - First, identify the morphology of the **normal** QRS complex and T wave for the animal.
> - This QRS–T morphology represents the normal depolarisation wave travelling *via the AV node*.
> - The QRS–T morphology of a ventricular ectopic complex is **different** from the normal QRS complex (that has passed via the AV node) and, therefore, must have arisen from within the ventricles.
> - Ventricular ectopic complexes are not associated with a preceding P wave (except by coincidence).

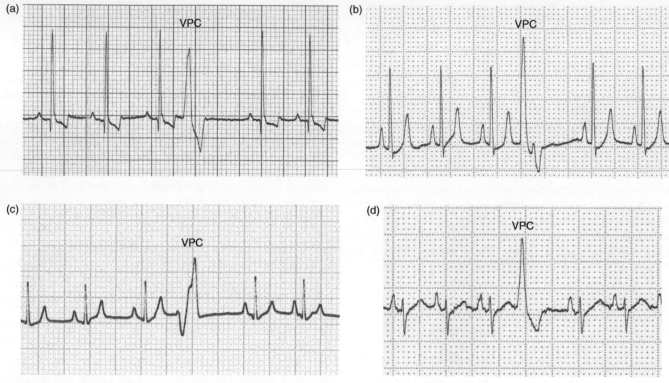

Figure 4.4 ECGs from three dogs (a, b, c) and a cat (d), each showing one ventricular ectopic complex in which the QRS morphology is not negative (cf. Figs 4.1 & 4.2), but exhibiting a different morphology. The fact that they are different from the morphology of the normal sinus QRS complexes is key to recognising that they are ventricular in origin (25 mm/s and 10 mm/mV).

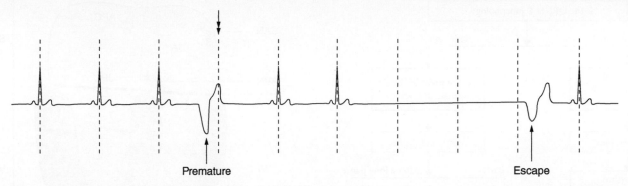

Premature

Escape

Figure 4.5 Illustration of a ventricular premature complex (the double-headed arrow indicates the time when the next normal sinus complex would have occurred) and a ventricular escape beat that occurred following a pause in the rhythm.

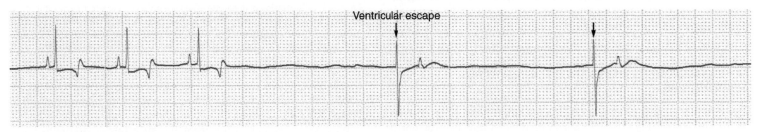

Ventricular escape

Figure 4.6 ECG from a WHWT dog, which has two ventricular escape complexes following a period of no electrical activity (i.e. sinus arrest, Chapter 7).

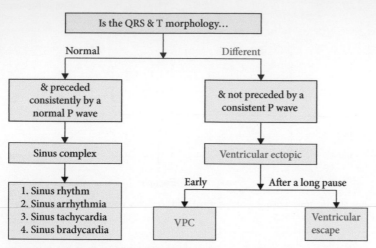

Figure 4.7 Flow chart summarising what we have described to this point. The important first step is to decide if the QRS and T morphology is 'normal' or 'different'. If different from normal, then the QRS complex is very likely to be a ventricular ectopic.

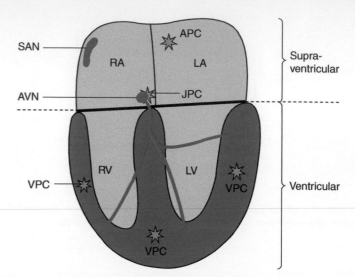

Figure 4.8 Illustration of the origin of supraventricular and ventricular ectopic complexes. SAN – sinoatrial node; AVN – atrioventricular node; APC – atrial premature complex; JPC – junctional premature complex; VPC – ventricular premature complex; RA – right atrium; LA – left atrium; RV – right ventricle; LV – left ventricle.

The morphology of an ectopic *supraventricular* depolarisation

Any ectopic stimuli arising above the ventricles are referred to as **supraventricular** (Fig. 4.8). These can be divided into two categories: (1) those occurring in the atrial muscle mass (atrial ectopics) and (2) those arising from within the AV node (**junctional** or **nodal** ectopics).

No matter where the supraventricular ectopics arise, they must travel down via the AV node and depolarise the ventricles normally. Thus, the morphology of the QRS complex associated with a supraventricular ectopic is normal,[2] that is the same as the QRS complex for a sinus complex. This means that the identification of a supraventricular ectopic

can be difficult. In the vast majority of cases, however, it occurs as a premature beat, and so it is primarily recognised by its premature timing (Figs 4.9 & 4.10).

Whether an ectopic arose from the atria (**atrial premature complex, APC**) or the AV node (referred to as a **junctional or nodal premature complex**) is of little practical importance in small animals until studying advanced ECGs. Additionally, in small animals, it does not often affect the management or treatment in the vast majority of cases. Therefore, the difference between atrial and junctional premature complexes will not be discussed here, and these are referred to by the broader term supraventricular premature complexes (SVPCs). However, it can be difficult to differentiate an early (normal) sinus complex from an APC, at times. As a general guideline:

---

[2] Except when there is aberrant conduction, see Chapter 10. However this is not common.

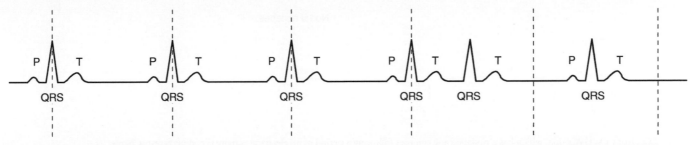

Figure 4.9 Illustration of a supraventricular premature complex (fifth beat), which is recognised mainly by its premature timing. The morphologies of the QRS and T are the same for both the sinus complexes and the SVPC because they both have passed through the AV node and depolarised the ventricles normally.

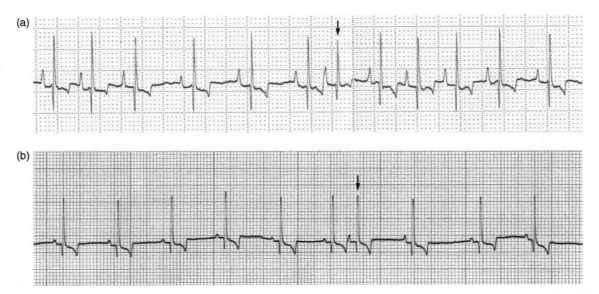

Figure 4.10 (a, b) ECGs from dogs showing supraventricular premature complexes (arrowed). Note that recognition is by the premature timing of the QRS and T, which have the same morphology as those of the normal sinus complexes (25 mm/s and 10 mm/mV).

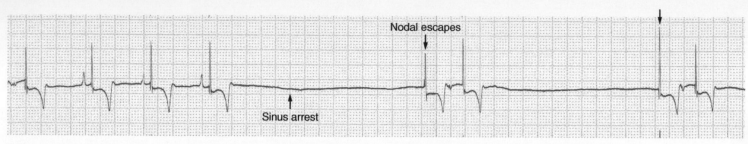

Figure 4.11 ECG from a WHWT dog, which has a nodal escape complex following a period of no electrical activity (i.e. sinus arrest (Chapter 7).

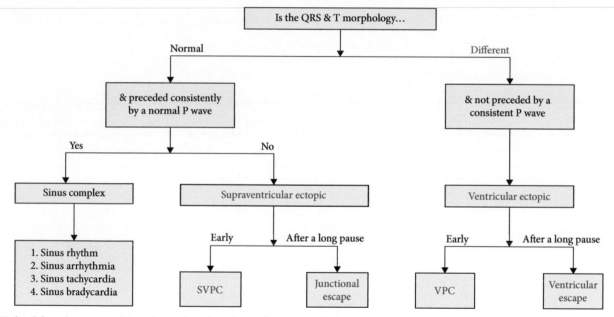

Figure 4.12 Updated flow chart summarising what we have described to this point, with the addition of supraventricular complexes. If a 'normal' complex is consistently preceded by a P wave, then this is a sinus complex; if not, then it is very likely to be a supraventricular complex.

(1) The P wave of an associated APC is usually of a different morphology compared to the normal sinus complexes.

(2) The P wave of an APC is typically so early that it becomes lost or superimposed in the preceding QRS and T waves, whereas the P wave of a normal sinus complex usually occurs after the preceding T wave.

A supraventricular ectopic complex can occur quickly (or early) and is, therefore, termed a **supraventricular** *premature* **complex** (SVPC) (Figs 4.9 & 4.10). If a supraventricular ectopic occurs after a pause (or with delay), then it is referred to as a **junctional** (or nodal) *escape* **complex** (Fig. 4.11).

The earlier flow chart (Fig 4.7) can now be updated to include SVPCs (Fig 4.12). When the shapes of the QRS and T complexes are normal, the next question is whether there are normal and consistent P waves are present or not. If not, then these are supraventricular ectopics. These can be classified as SVPCs when their timing is premature, and as junctional escapes when they occur after a long pause.

Key points

- Any ectopic stimuli arising above the ventricles are referred to as **supraventricular**.
- Wherever supraventricular ectopics arise, they must travel down via the AV node and depolarise the ventricles normally.
- The morphology of the QRS complex and T wave associated with a supraventricular ectopic is the **same** as that of a normal sinus complex.
- It is primarily recognised by its premature timing.

Compensatory and non-compensatory pauses explained

This is terminology that is mentioned sometimes, and it is probably best to explain what it means (Fig 4.13).

A full compensatory pause. When there is a VPC during a normal sinus rhythm, the ventricles become refractory to the normal sinus node-generated depolarisation wave. The sinus node continues to fire undisturbed at its regular rate, so the next depolarisation of the ventricles occurs after the ventricles have repolarised following the VPC. But since the VPC was premature, there is a longer than normal R–R duration between the VPC and the next sinus complex. The duration from the sinus complex before the VPC until the one after the VPC is equivalent to two R–R intervals. This longer pause after the VPC is termed a full compensatory pause (Fig 4.5). The VPCs illustrated in Figs 4.2a, 4.2b, 4.4b, 4.4d, and 4.4 all meet these criteria (but not those in Fig. 4.4a and 4.4c).

A non-compensatory pause. When there is an APC, it depolarises the SA node and resets the rate at that time point, that is, the interval from the APC to the following sinus complex is equivalent to the normal R–R duration. Consequently, the duration from the sinus complex before the APC until the sinus complex after the APC is less than the equivalent of two R–R intervals. This is referred to as a non-compensatory pause. This works for the second SVPC in Fig. 4.9 but less so for the first complex.

A full compensatory pause is considered to more likely follow a VPC, and a non-compensatory pause to follow an APC. However, it is now known that following a VPC, there can be retrograde conduction up the AV node in animals, which has the potential to reset the SA node; additionally, SPVCs may not reset the SA node and thus produce a full compensatory pause. This terminology is therefore now considered less reliable.

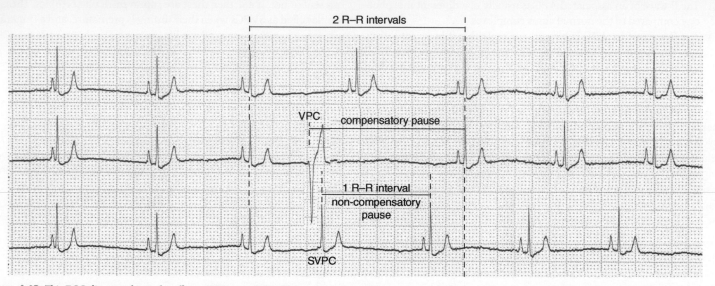

Figure 4.13 This ECG diagram shows the effect a VPC or an SVPC has on the timing of the next normal sinus complex. The VPC is followed by a full compensatory pause, whereas the SVPC resets the sinus node and therefore is followed by a non-compensatory pause. However, this criterion to differentiate VPCs and SVPCs is now considered unreliable.

5 • Ventricular arrhythmias

This chapter discusses the electrocardiographic features, as well as the clinical findings, of the more common ventricular arrhythmias. Please note that the clinical significance and treatment of these arrhythmias are discussed in Chapter 13.

Ventricular arrhythmias

Ventricular premature complexes

Ventricular premature complexes (VPCs) are a common finding in dogs and cats. VPCs arise from an ectopic focus or foci within the ventricular myocardium. Depolarisation, therefore, occurs in an abnormal direction through the myocardium, and the impulse conducts from cell to cell as described in Chapter 4.

ECG characteristics

The QRS complex morphology is different from normal (abnormal) and traditionally described as wide and bizarre in shape, that is, unlike a QRS that would have arisen via the AV node. It is usually:

- Abnormal (bizarre) in shape (i.e. different from the normal QRS).
- Wide (prolonged) – QRS duration is typically prolonged by ~50%.

- The T wave of a VPC is often large and opposite in direction to the QRS.
- P waves may or may not be identified – if they are seen, they are unrelated to the QRS complex, except by coincidence.

Examples of single VPCs in dogs and cats are shown in Figs 5.1a, b, & c and 5.2a & b. Because a VPC occurs prematurely, a normal sinus depolarisation arriving at the AV node will meet the ventricles when they are refractory; thus, the P wave is usually hidden by the ventricular premature complex (Fig 5.3a, b).

Clinical findings

Occasional premature beats will sound like a '**tripping in the rhythm**'. Depending upon how early the beat occurs – the 'extra' premature beat may be heard, or it might be 'silent' (in which case it would sound like a pause in the rhythm or a dropped beat). There will be little or no pulse associated with the premature beat, which is termed a **pulse deficit**. If the premature beats are more frequent, the tripping in the rhythm will start to make the heart rhythm sound more irregular. With very frequent premature beats, the heart rhythm can sound quite chaotic, and with a pulse deficit for each premature beat, the pulse rate will be much slower than the heart rate.

Small Animal ECGs: An Introductory Guide, Third Edition. Mike Martin.
© 2015 John Wiley & Sons, Ltd. Published 2015 by John Wiley & Sons, Ltd.

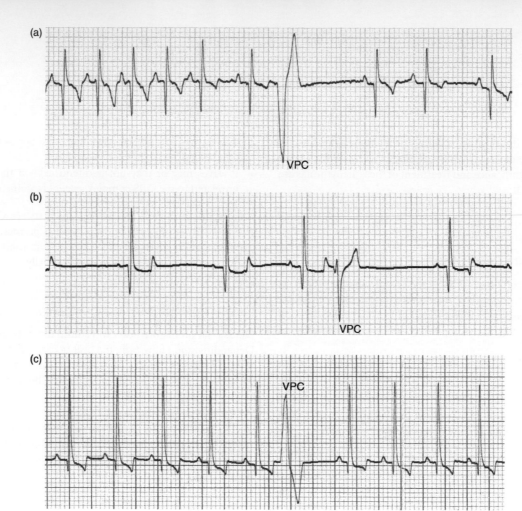

Figure 5.1 (a–c) ECGs from three dogs, each showing a single VPC (25 mm/s and 10 mm/mV).

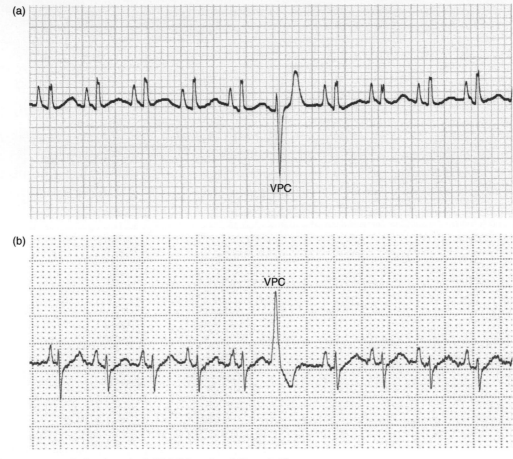

Figure 5.2 (a, b) ECGs from two cats, each showing a single VPC (25 mm/s and 10 mm/mV).

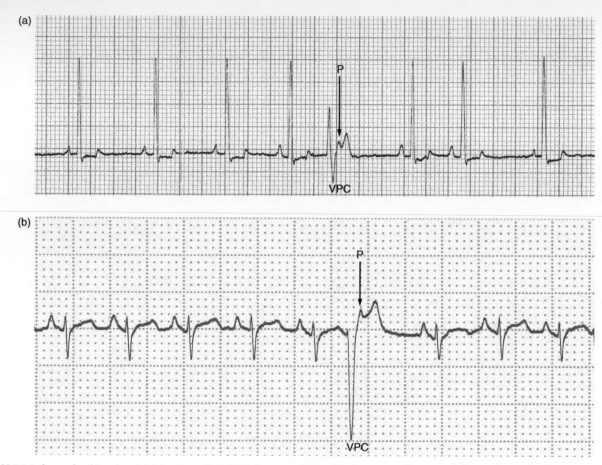

Figure 5.3 (a, b) ECGs from a dog (a) and a cat (b) showing a single VPC; however, additionally, there is a small positive deflection (just before the T wave) consistent with a P wave (arrowed). When the normal sinus depolarisation arrived at the AV node, the ventricles were still refractory.

Ventricular tachycardia

A run of four[1] or more VPCs is termed a ventricular tachycardia (VT) (Fig 5.4a–e). In the vast majority of cases, VT is fairly uniform and regular; however, occasionally, it can be multiform (or polymorphic) (Fig. 5.5a & b). The duration of VT can additionally be described as paroxysmal VT when it is very short (Fig. 5.4b), as non-sustained VT (Fig. 5.4c) when it does not exceed 30 seconds or as sustained VT (Fig. 5.4d, e) when it is does exceed 30 seconds.

ECG characteristics

The morphology is of a sequence of VPCs, typically at a rate >180/min.

Clinical findings

During a sustained VT, the heart rhythm will usually sound fairly regular (i.e. potentially unremarkable) – pulses will probably be palpable, but reduced in strength, becoming weaker with faster heart rates. If there is a break or interruption to the VT, then this irregularity will be heard. During a sustained VT, the systolic blood pressure is usually low.

---

[1] The definition of how many of VPCs in sequence constitutes a VT is variable and ranges from 3 to 6 complexes. It is not particularly important in a clinical setting, however, because three VPCs in sequence are more commonly referred to as a triplet; VT is defined in this book as a run of four or more VPCs.

Terminology of ventricular arrhythmias

The electrocardiographic interpretation of arrhythmias due to ectopia requires an understanding of the terminology used. If this is accomplished, interpretation becomes relatively easy.

Ventricular ectopic complexes may be classified by the following:

(1) *Timing.* Ventricular ectopic complexes that occur before the next normal complex would have been due are termed **ventricular premature complexes (VPCs)** (Figs 5.1, 5.2 & 5.3), and those that occur following a pause such as a period of sinus arrest or in complete heart block are termed **ventricular escapes** (Fig. 4.6).

(2) *Numbers in Sequence.* VPCs may occur singly (as in Figs 5.1, 5.2 & 5.3), in couplets (or pairs) (Fig 5.5a) or in triplets (Fig 5.5b). Runs of four[1] or more are referred to as a **ventricular tachycardia (VT)** (Fig 5.4a–e).

(3) *Frequency.* The number of VPCs in a tracing may vary from occasional to very frequent. When there is a set ratio such as one sinus complex to one ventricular ectopic, it is termed **ventricular bigeminy** (Fig 5.6a), and one ectopic to two sinus complexes is termed **ventricular trigeminy** (Fig 5.6b). If a single VPC occurs in between two sinus complexes, without disturbing the sinus rhythm, it is termed an **interpolated VPC** (Fig 5.7).

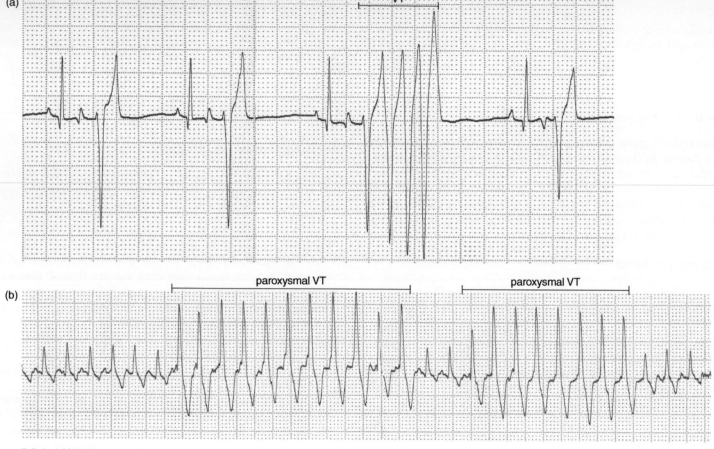

(a)

VT

(b)

paroxysmal VT   paroxysmal VT

Figure 5.4 (a & b) ECGs tracings from two dogs showing differing durations of ventricular tachycardia (VT). Four or more VPCs (a) constitutes a VT and paroxysmal VT is of short duration (b).

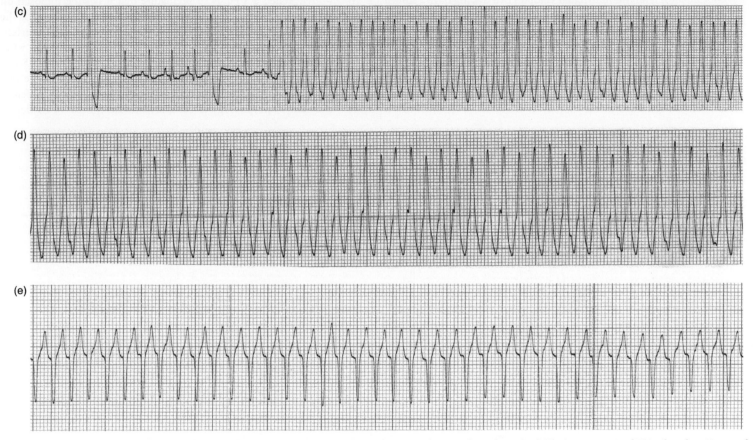

Figure 5.4 (c–e) ECGs tracings from two dogs (c & d) and a cat (e) showing differing durations of ventricular tachycardia (VT). A non-sustained VT is less than 30 seconds (c) and sustained VT is considered longer than 30 seconds (d & e).

(4) *Morphology.* If all the ventricular ectopics in a tracing have a similar morphology, they are referred to as **uniform** or **monomorphic** (Fig 5.4a–e) and those with different shapes are termed **multiform** or **polymorphic** (Fig. 5.8a & b).

(5) *Duration of VT* can additionally be described as **paroxysmal VT** (Fig 5.4b) when it is short, **non-sustained VT** (Fig 5.4c) when it does not exceed 30 s (which is a nominal value) or **sustained VT** (5.4 d, e) when it exceeds 30 s.

(6) *R-on-T.* When a VPC is so premature that it is superimposed on the T wave of the preceding complex (sinus or ectopic), that is the ventricles are depolarised before they have completely repolarised (from the preceding contraction), this is termed R-on-T (Fig. 5.9).

(7) *Fusion Complexes.* Occasionally, a normal sinus complex QRS will occur at the same time as a VPC, resulting in fusion of the two wave fronts. A **fusion complex** is seen on an ECG with a different QRS and T morphology as compared to the typical VPCs due to

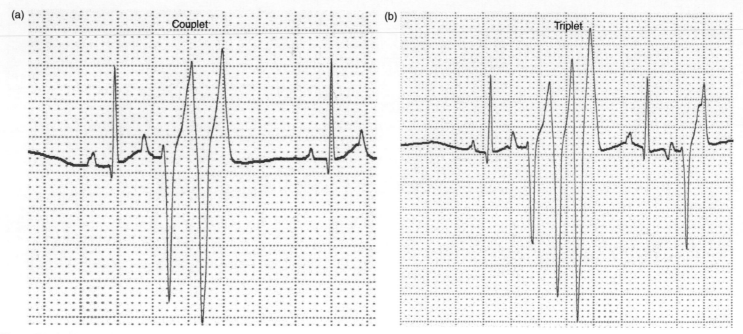

Figure 5.5 (a, b) ECGs from two dogs showing grouping of VPCs; these are termed: a couplet (a) and a triplet (b).

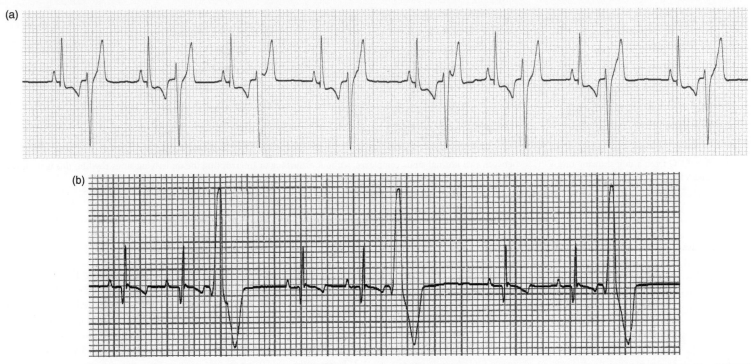

Figure 5.6 (a) ECG from a CKCS dog with MVD showing sinus complexes alternating with ventricular premature complexes; this is termed ventricular bigeminy. (b) ECG from a Boxer dog with a urinary tract condition, showing two sinus complexes alternating with ventricular premature complexes; this is termed ventricular trigeminy. In both ECGs, the VPCs are all of the same morphology; thus, the VPCs are termed uniform. Fig 5.6b courtesy of Paul Wotton.

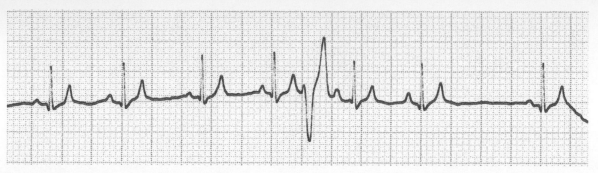

Figure 5.7 ECG from a dog showing one VPC in-between two normal sinus complexes, without disturbing or interrupting the underlying sinus rhythm; this is termed an interpolated VPC.

the merging of the QRS and T of the sinus complex and VPC. Usually, the complexes in combination tend to cancel each other out (i.e. neutralise the deflections) and the QRS is much smaller in comparison to the typical VPCs (Fig 5.10a, b).

A word about terminology

Understanding ECGs is as much about learning the vocabulary as it is about recognising different ECG complexes; it is like a language in itself. However, in order to have conversations with colleagues or seek advice from experts, you need to be able to speak the language and use the correct terminology; otherwise, communication will be difficult.

Ventricular fibrillation (VF)

Depolarisation waves occur chaotically and rapidly throughout the ventricles (Fig 5.11). This is nearly always a terminal event associated with cardiac arrest. There is no significant coordinated contraction to produce any cardiac output. If the heart is visualised or palpated, fine irregular movements of the ventricles are evident (likened to a 'can of worms'). Ventricular fibrillation (VF) is usually preceded by a very fast VT, typically with R-on-T.

ECG characteristics

The ECG shows **coarse** (larger) or **fine** (smaller) rapid, irregular and bizarre movement with no normal waves or complexed (Fig. 5.12).

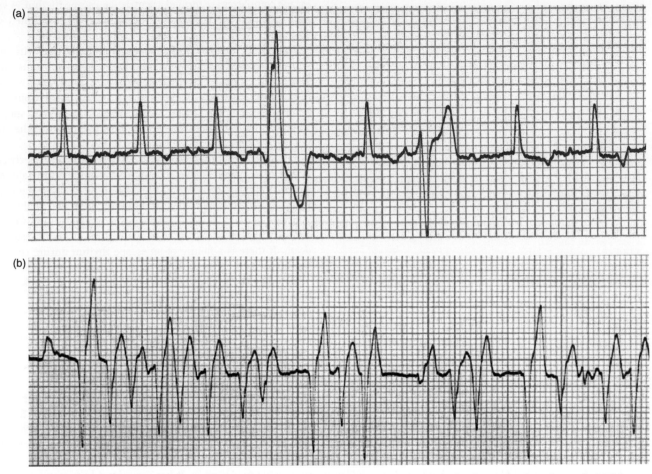

(a)

(b)

Figure 5.8 (a, b) ECGs from two dogs showing multiple VPCs on the tracing, with different shapes; these are termed multimorphic (or polymorphic) VPCs.

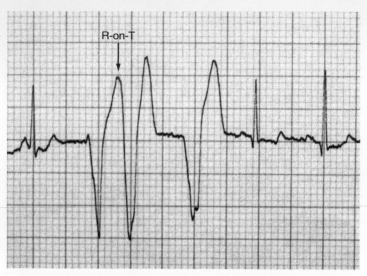

Figure 5.9 ECGs from a dog showing R-on-T, the second of the VPCs commences on the T wave of the preceding VPC.

Clinical findings

No heart sounds are heard. No pulse is palpable.

Ventricular escape rhythms

When the dominant pacemaker tissue (usually, the SA node) fails to discharge for a long period, pacemaker tissue with a slower intrinsic rate may then discharge, that is, it 'escapes' the control of the SA node. An escape beat that arises from the ventricles (i.e. a ventricular ectopic) is termed a ventricular escape complex (Fig 5.13a). A series of ventricular escape complexes are termed a ventricular escape rhythm. A ventricular escape rhythm differs from a VT in that it is very slow (often <60/min), typically 30–40/min.

Ventricular escape rhythms are commonly seen in association with bradyarrhythmias (e.g. sinus bradycardia, sinus arrest, AV block) (Chapter 7). Escape complexes are sometimes referred to as rescue beats, because if they did not occur, death would be imminent. Since they are rescue beats, they should not be suppressed by medications. Treatment should be directed towards the underlying bradyarrhythmia.

If no escape rhythm developed, that is, there was no electrical activity of any kind, then it is termed **asystole** (Chapter 7). The absence of any electrical activity would result in a 'flatline' on the ECG tracing. It would not be dissimilar to sustained sinus arrest if no escape rhythm developed. A period of asystole would result in syncope; however, if there was no return of electrical activity or escape rhythm, it would result in sudden death. If there is a failure of an escape rhythm during complete heart block, that is, there are P waves but no QRS complexes, then it is termed **ventricular standstill** (Fig 5.13b) (Chapter 7). Heart block with a period of ventricular standstill would result in syncope, but if there was no return of electrical activity or escape rhythm, it would result in sudden death.

Accelerated idioventricular rhythm (AIVR)

Accelerated idioventricular rhythm (AIVR) is a descriptive term for a ventricular ectopic rhythm with a rate in between the rates of a ventricular escape rhythm (often 30–50/min in dog and 90–110/min in cats, Fig 5.14), and a VT (often >180/min). It occurs when a focus that should normally be suppressed increases at a rate faster than that of the sinus node or AV node. It has sometimes been given the nickname a

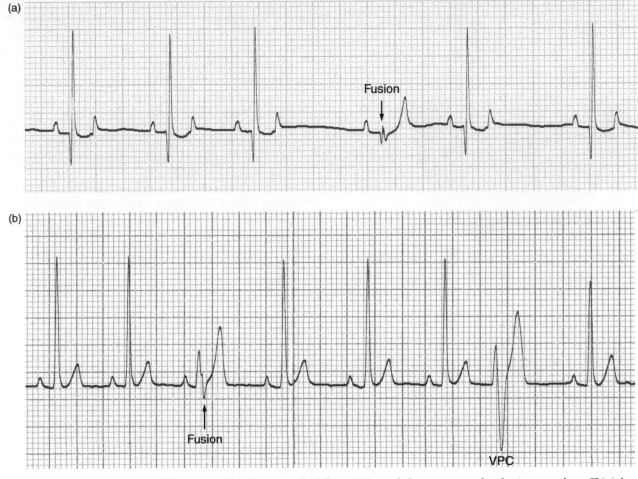

Figure 5.10 (a, b) In (a), the fourth complex (which is preceded by a P wave) is of a different QRS morphology as compared to the sinus complexes. This is because there was a VPC at the same moment, and the two QRS complexes thus cancelled each other out, leaving a small bizarre deflection: this is termed a fusion complex (arrowed). In (b), the third complex is a 'fusion' of the QRS and T between a normal sinus complex and a VPC (second last complex).

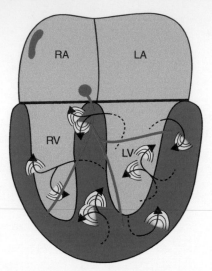

'slow ventricular tachycardia'. There is overlap in the rates for AIVR and VT, but in general, the upper limit is considered to be around 180–220/min, although AIVR or VT should not be diagnosed on the basis of rate alone.

AIVR is generally an intermittent and transient rhythm (although it may persist for some days) that is well tolerated and rarely causes haemodynamic compromise or hypotension and does not require treatment. It is generally considered a benign rhythm that is self-limiting and is most unlikely to result in death and usually resolves naturally after the inciting cause has resolved. Rarely would AIVR degenerate into VT or VF. In contrast, VT often has a poorer prognosis and is typically associated with hypotension and pallor.

The mechanism of AIVR appears to be related to the enhanced automaticity in the His–Purkinje fibres and/or myocardium (vagal excess and decreased sympathetic activity), that is, an enhanced ventricular ectopic rhythm. When the enhanced automaticity in the His–Purkinje fibres or myocardium surpasses that of the sinus node, AIVR manifests as the dominant rhythm of the heart. Sinus bradycardia may facilitate the appearance of AIVR.

Figure 5.11 Diagram illustrating the wavelet theory for ventricular fibrillation (VF). VF initially consists of large wavelets (coarse VF), which progress over a short period of time to a greater number of smaller wavelets (fine VF).

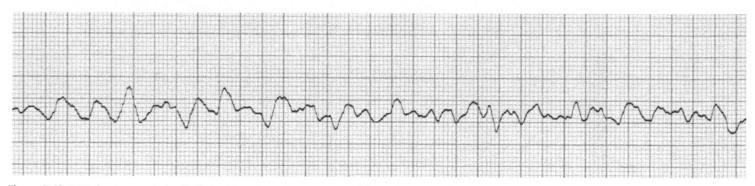

Figure 5.12 ECG showing ventricular fibrillation. Note the random movement of the ECG tracing and absence of anything recognisable. (25 mm/s and 10 mm/mV).

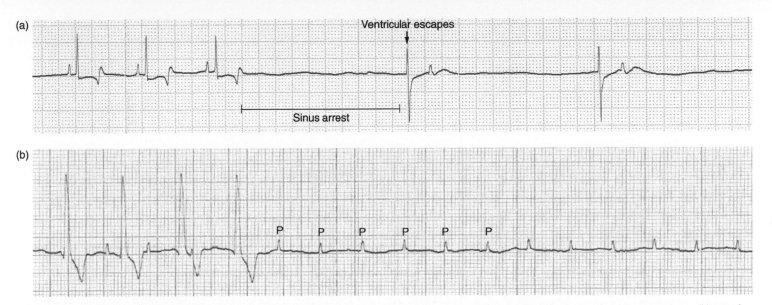

Figure 5.13 (a) ECG from a WHWT showing an initial three sinus complexes, then a pause of sinus arrest, following which there are ventricular escape beats. (b) ECG from a Weimaraner with complete heart block, initially with a nodal escape rhythm; however, then an absence of the escape rhythm is absent, which is termed ventricular standstill (this seems to be a common mechanism of collapse in dogs with heart block).

ECG characteristics

There are two competing rhythms present – the underlying sinus rhythm and the enhanced ventricular ectopic rhythm – which are often at similar rates (Fig 5.14).

- The ventricular rhythm manifests when the underlying sinus rhythm slows down (to less than the ventricular rhythm) or when the ventricular rhythm accelerates above the sinus rhythm.
- Onset is typically gradual, starting with either a ventricular escape beat or a fusion beat or a late premature beat, and may often occur during a slowing phase of the sinus rhythm.
- Termination is often gradual and may end with a fusion beat or speeding up of the sinus rhythm.
- Slow onset and termination of AIVR is considered important when differentiating it from VT, which is more often associated with sudden onset and termination.
- The ventricular rhythm can be fairly regular, often intermittently transient and interspersed with normal sinus complexes, and a little faster than the underlying sinus rhythm (resulting in AV dissociation).
- The ventricular ectopic rhythm typically has a rate of 100–200/min, but within a range from 50/min up to 220/min.

41

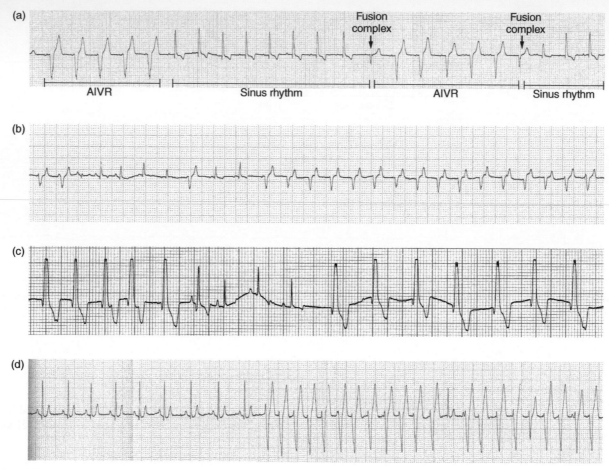

Figure 5.14 (a) ECG from a Boxer with endocarditis with AIVR. Note the two competing rhythms present – the underlying sinus rhythm and the enhanced ventricular ectopic rhythm – which are at similar rates. The ventricular rhythm is not fast enough to be termed a ventricular tachycardia. Also note the two fusion complexes (arrowed). (b) ECG from a Labrador with a splenic mass. There is an underlying sinus rhythm with an AIVR (at 160/min). (c) ECG from a 6-year-old Labrador while under general anaesthesia for orthopaedic surgery (courtesy of Anne French). (d) ECG from an old Labrador with a splenic mass. Again, note the two rhythms. The ventricular rhythm is 200/min here, and in this case, it can be difficult to decide if it is AIVR or a ventricular tachycardia.

- The morphology of the ventricular ectopics is usually uniform (monomorphic) and mostly regular. A polymorphic ventricular rhythm is uncommon with AIVR.
- Because there are two underlying competing rhythms, ventricular depolarisation can sometimes coincide, leading to fusion beats, particularly at the onset or termination of the rhythm (Fig 5.14a).

Clinical findings

The rhythm is irregular because of the intermingling of sinus beats with the AIVR. The heart rate is often not particularly fast, being within the range of 100–200/min.

Note

It is important to measure the blood pressure with any arrhythmia, but more so in differentiating between AIVR and VT. A BP <100 mmHg systolic would be considered low (<90 mmHg is very low). A blood pressure >120 mmHg systolic would be considered good in dogs with an arrhythmia. If the animal becomes hypotensive, then consider if the ventricular rhythm truly is a VT, or could there be a concurrent medical condition causing the hypotension.

6 • Supraventricular arrhythmias

This chapter discusses the electrocardiographic features, as well as the clinical findings, of the more common supraventricular arrhythmias. Please note that the clinical significance and treatment of these arrhythmias are discussed in Chapter 14.

Supraventricular arrhythmias

Supraventricular premature complexes

Supraventricular premature complexes (SVPCs) arise from an ectopic focus or foci above the ventricles, that is, in either the atria, the AV node or the bundle of His. The ventricles are then depolarised normally, producing a normally shaped QRS complex with a normal duration.

ECG characteristics

QRS–T complexes, which have a normal morphology, are seen to occur prematurely (Fig. 6.1). The ECG features are:

- Normal QRS morphology
  - There can be a minor variation from 'normal', but usually within 90% of being normal
- QRS duration is <0.07 seconds.[1]

[1] Except when there is aberrant conduction, see Chapter 11.

Small Animal ECGs: An Introductory Guide, Third Edition. Mike Martin.
© 2015 John Wiley & Sons, Ltd. Published 2015 by John Wiley & Sons, Ltd.

- QRS complexes are seen to occur prematurely.
- P waves may or may not be identified.
- If P waves are seen, they are usually of an abnormal morphology (i.e. non-sinus) and the P–R interval will differ from a normal sinus complex.

Clinical findings

On auscultation, when there is a premature beat, it is not possible to distinguish between a supraventricular and a ventricular premature beat (Chapter 4). Occasional premature beats will sound like a '**tripping in the rhythm**', with little or no pulse associated with the premature beat (pulse deficit). If the premature beats are more frequent, the tripping in the rhythm will start to make the heart rhythm sound more irregular. With very frequent premature beats, the heart rhythm can sound quite chaotic, and with a pulse deficit for each premature beat, the pulse rate will be much slower than the heart rate.

> **Note**
>
> While the clinical findings on examination of a patient are discussed here, the clinical significance of tachyarrhythmias is discussed in Chapter 14.

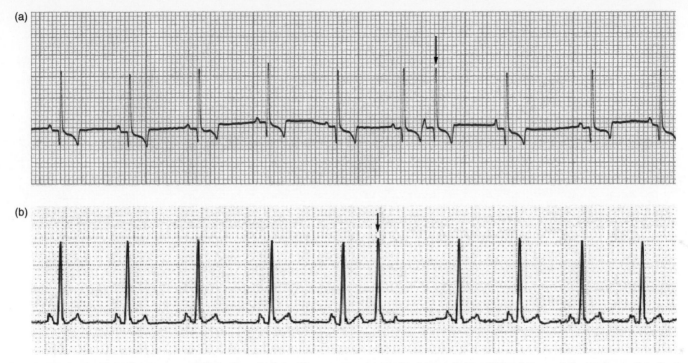

Figure 6.1 (a) ECG from a CKCS showing an underlying sinus rhythm with one premature complex (arrowed). The QRS and T morphology is 'normal', indicating this is a supraventricular complex (SVPC). It looks like there is a P wave preceding this SVPC, superimposed on the preceding T wave. (b) ECG from a Border Terrier showing an underlying sinus arrhythmia with a premature SVPC (arrowed) (25 mm/s and 10 mm/mV). ECG tracing courtesy of Jo Dukes McEwan.

Supraventricular tachycardia

A run of four[2] or more SVPCs is termed a **supraventricular tachycardia (SVT)**; it is usually a rate in excess of 200/min, but typically 250–350/min, although it can be as high as 400/min in dogs and regular (Fig. 6.2). SVT needs to be distinguished from a sinus tachycardia, which often exceeds 200/min and can reach in excess of 250/min (in dogs).

---

[2] The definition of the number of SVPCs in sequence constitutes an SVT is variable and ranges from 3 to 6 complexes. It is not particularly important in a clinical setting, however, because three SVPCs in sequence are more commonly referred to as a triplet, SVT is defined in this book as a run of four or more of SVPCs.

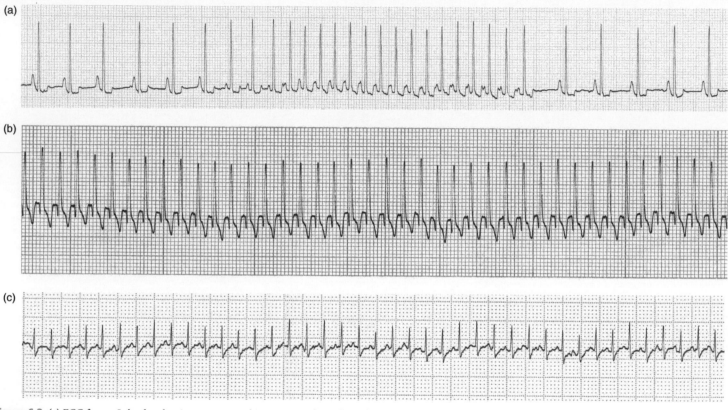

Figure 6.2 (a) ECG from a Labrador showing a paroxysmal supraventricular tachycardia at 260/min (25 mm/s and 10 mm/mV). (b) ECG from a Bulldog showing a sustained supraventricular tachycardia (SVT) at 320/min. No normal sinus complexes are seen (25 mm/s and 10 mm/mV). (c) ECG from a cat showing a sustained supraventricular tachycardia at 340/min. No normal sinus complexes are seen (25 mm/s and 5 mm/mV).

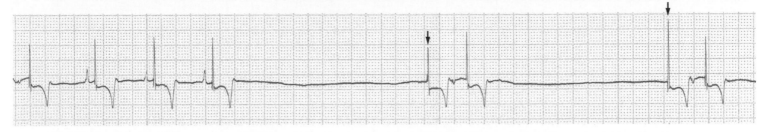

Figure 6.3 ECG from a WHWT with sinus arrest. Following the long pauses, there are junctional escape complexes (arrowed) (25 mm/s and 10 mm/mV).

ECG characteristics

The morphology is of a sequence of SVPCs and typically at a rate >250/min.

Clinical findings

During a sustained SVT, the heart rhythm will sound fairly regular – pulses will probably be palpable, but weak or reduced in strength, becoming weaker with faster heart rates. Sometimes, only alternate heart beats produce a pulse (pulsus alternans); thus, the pulse rate is half the heart rate. During a sustained SVT, the systolic blood pressure will be low or low-normal.

Terminology of supraventricular arrhythmias

The electrocardiographic interpretation of arrhythmias due to ectopia requires an understanding of the terminology used. If this is accomplished, interpretation becomes relatively easy.

Supraventricular ectopic complexes may be classified by the following:

(1) *Timing.* Supraventricular ectopic complexes that occur before the next normal complex (Fig. 6.1) would have been due are termed supraventricular premature complexes (SVPCs), and those that occur following a pause such as a period of sinus arrest (Fig. 6.3) or in complete heart block are termed **junctional escapes**.

(2) *Number of ectopics.* SVPCs may occur singly, in pairs or in triplets (Fig. 6.4), and a run of four or more is referred to as an **supraventricular tachycardia (SVT)**.

(3) *Duration of SVT* can additionally be described as **paroxysmal SVT** when it is very short (Fig. 6.2a), **non-sustained SVT** when it does not exceed 30 s (which is a nominal value) or **sustained SVT** when it exceeds 30 s (Fig. 6.2b, c).

Narrow QRS complex tachycardia

This is a descriptive term used to describe any fast rhythm in which the QRS complexes are narrow and fairly normal in appearance, and it may also include sinus tachycardia (when the P waves are not clearly discernible) or even atrial fibrillation (AF). It is used to differentiate it from a broad QRS complex tachycardia (Chapter 5). An SVT can be described as a narrow QRS complex tachycardia when the QRS duration is normal (<0.07 s).

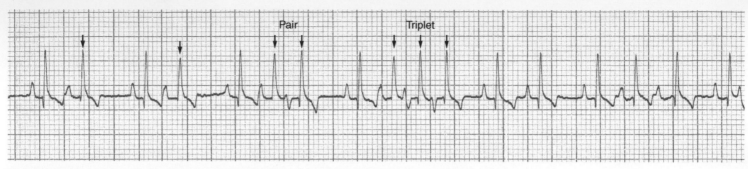

Figure 6.4 ECG from a dog showing frequent SVPCs in singles, pairs and triplets (arrowed) (25 mm/s and 10 mm/mV).

Tip

Differentiation between supraventricular and ventricular arrhythmias

Supraventricular	*Ventricular*
'Normal': narrow QRS complex.	'Different': wide and bizarre QRS complex
Heart rate often 250–400/min	Heart rate often 180–300/min
Absence of fusion beats.	Presence of fusion beats

Atrioventricular dissociation

Atrioventricular (AV) dissociation describes the situation where the atria and ventricles are driven by independent pacemakers at equal or nearly equal rates. This arrhythmia is also sometimes termed **isorhythmic AV dissociation**. The mechanism of action of this rhythm is not clearly understood, and there are a number of hypotheses, one of which is the presence of an AV nodal tachycardia that virtually matches the sinus node rate. It is considered a benign rhythm of little or no clinical significance, but when there is loss of mechanical atrioventricular coordination (i.e. when atrial contraction does not precede ventricular contraction), there can be a small fall in blood pressure. AV dissociation seems to be more common in Labradors than in other breeds and may be seen in dogs that are a little 'stressed' or during anaesthesia. It seems to be rare in cats.

ECG characteristics

The P waves and QRS complexes are independent of each other, with P waves appearing to drift gradually back and forth across the QRS complexes producing a variation in the PR intervals (Fig. 6.5a & b).

The P waves may occur before, during or after the QRS complex, but usually do not 'move' through the T wave or ST segment.

The heart rate is usually normal or slightly fast, and the variation in rate between the two pacemakers is very small (in contrast to complete AV block in which the ventricular rate is significantly slower and different from the P waves).

Clinical findings

In most cases, the heart rhythm will sound fairly normal and the pulse should match the heart rate. Occasionally, there may be a 'tripping in the rhythm' associated with the timing of the AV nodal tachycardia or re-capture of sinus rhythm.

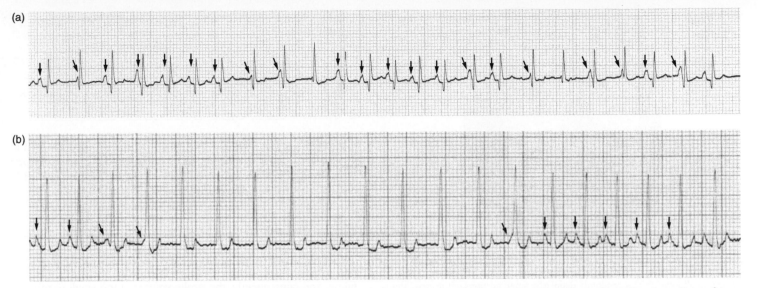

Figure 6.5 (a, b) ECGs from two Labradors with AV dissociation. Note how the P waves (arrowed) seem to drift in and out of the QRS complexes; there is one P wave for every QRS, but there is not a constant P–R interval (25 mm/s and 10 mm/mV).

Atrial fibrillation

AF is probably one of the most common and important arrhythmias seen in small animals. Since AF originates above the ventricles, it can also be classified as a supraventricular arrhythmia.

AF in animals most commonly occurs as a consequence of atrial dilation and more usually in larger breed dogs. Once AF develops in animals, it is nearly always permanent and continuous. However, occasionally in large or giant breed dogs, AF can occur without the presence of the underlying structural heart disease or abnormally dilated atria; this is referred to as **lone AF**. Occasionally, on Holter recordings, there can be intermittent periods of AF that may last from minutes

to hours; this is termed **paroxysmal AF**. This is rare in dogs and cats, although more common in humans and in horses.

In AF, multiple wavelets of electrical activity randomly circulate throughout the atria (Fig. 6.6). Many hundreds of depolarisation waves, per minute, arrive at the AV node randomly; however, not all are conducted as many arrive at the AV node when it is still refractory (i.e. many are blocked). This results in a random and chaotic ventricular depolarisation. Thus, the ventricular response rate and rhythm (to the fibrillating atria) creates a fast and chaotic sounding heart on auscultation. The ventricular rate (heart rate) during AF is dictated by the ability of the AV node to conduct the impulses, which is influenced by autonomic tone. AV nodal conduction is enhanced by sympathetic

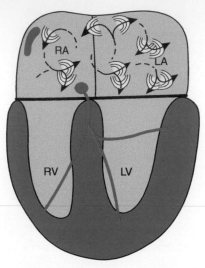

Figure 6.6 Diagram illustrating the wavelet theory for atrial fibrillation. Note the multiple small wavelets that randomly depolarise small portions of the atria. This is easiest to sustain when the atria are large such as in giant-breed dogs or animals in which there is atrial dilation.

activity; thus, the ventricular response rate is faster than when there is a high vagal tone.

ECG characteristics

The QRS complexes have a normal morphology (similarly to SVPCs described earlier) and occur at a normal-to-fast rate (Fig. 6.7). The ECG features are:

- Normal QRS morphology.[3]
- The R–R interval is irregular and chaotic (this is easier to hear on auscultation).
- The QRS complexes often vary in amplitude.

---

[3] Except when there is bundle branch block (see Chapter 11).

- There are no consistent and recognisable P waves preceding the QRS complex.

> **Tip**
>
> As a guideline: Supraventricular QRS morphology[3] + Chaotic R–R intervals + Absence of P waves = AF

- Sometimes, fine irregular movements of the baseline are seen as a result of the atrial fibrillation waves – referred to as '**f waves;** however, these are frequently indistinguishable from the baseline artefact (e.g. muscle tremor) in small animals.

Clinical findings

The heart rhythm on auscultation sounds chaotic and usually quite fast. Left ventricular filling time is very variable, often too short for adequate filling, and consequently, the stroke volume is too small to produce a palpable pulse for many beats. Hence, the pulse rate is often half the heart rate, hence there is a 50% pulse deficit, especially when the heart rate with atrial fibrillation is fast. A fast and chaotic heart on auscultation with a 50% pulse deficit is characteristic of AF. However, very frequent premature beats (ventricular or supraventricular) can mimic this.

> **What is a pulse deficit?**
>
> If an auscultated heart beat fails to produce a palpable pulse, it is termed a pulse deficit. This can occur with premature beats or arrhythmias associated with very early beats. This is common with ventricular and supraventricular arrhythmias and, in particular, AF. If a premature or early beat is auscultated, but does not produce sufficient stroke volume to generate a palpable pulse, this is a pulse deficit. If premature or early beats are particularly common such as occurs with AF, the pulses deficits are frequent. Typically in AF, there is often >50% pulse deficit.

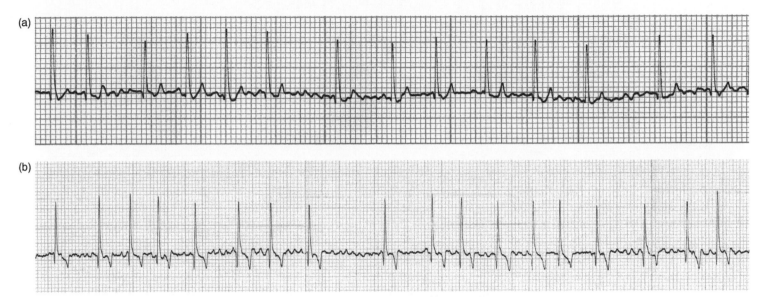

Figure 6.7 ECGs from four dogs and one cat with atrial fibrillation (AF). All show a supraventricular rhythm that is chaotic, without preceding P waves: which is consistent with AF. (a) ECG from a Bull Mastiff with AF with a heart rate of 150/min. This dog had no underlying heart disease, which is consistent with 'lone AF'. (b) ECG from an Irish Setter with AF with a heart rate of 130/min. This dog had a very dilated left atrium secondary to mitral valve disease (MVD).

51

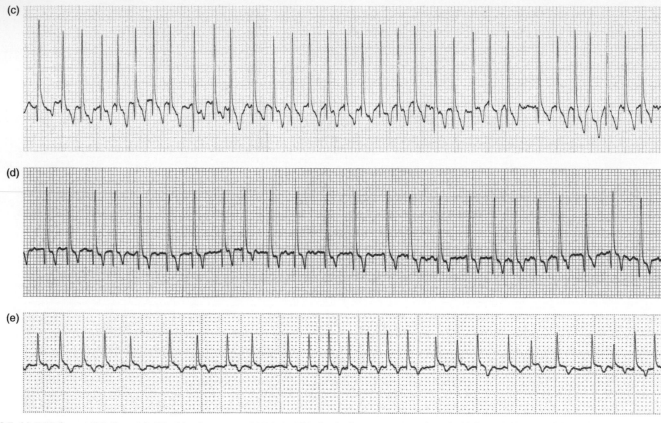

Figure 6.7 (c) ECG from a Shih Tzu with AF with a heart rate of 230/min. This dog had severe MVD and marked left atrial dilation. (d) ECG from a GSD with AF with a heart rate of 190/min. This dog had dilated cardiomyopathy. (e) ECG from a cat with AF with a heart rate of 240/min. This cat had massively dilated atria secondary to restrictive cardiomyopathy. (All tracings recorded at 25 mm/s and 10 mm/mV).

Junctional escape rhythms

While escapes beats are commonly ventricular in origin (see Ventricular escape rhythm in Chapter 5), an escape beat can also arise from the AV node or the bundle of His. In this case, it is termed a junctional (or nodal) escape complex. A series of nodal escape complexes are termed a junctional (or nodal) escape rhythm.

Junctional escapes are fairly normal in shape (the same as a supraventricular ectopic); see Fig. 6.8. A nodal escape rhythm differs from an SVT in that it is very slow, typically 50–70/min in dogs. Like ventricular escape rhythms, a nodal escape rhythm is usually seen in association with bradyarrhythmias (e.g. sinus bradycardia, sinus arrest, AV block, atrial standstill).

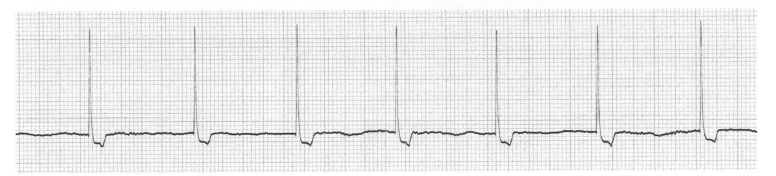

Figure 6.8 ECG from a miniature Schnauzer with atrial standstill and a nodal escape rhythm at 60/min (25 mm/s and 10 mm/mV).

7 • Abnormalities in the conduction system

This chapter discusses the electrocardiographic features, as well as the clinical findings, of the more common arrhythmias due to abnormalities in the conduction system. Please note that the clinical significance and treatment of these arrhythmias are discussed in Chapter 15.

Abnormalities in the conduction system are associated with faults in either the generation of the impulse from the SA node or the abnormalities in conduction through the specialised conduction tissue, that is, the AV node, bundle of His and Purkinje system. Generally, these faults result in arrhythmias in which the heart rhythm is slow, and are often termed bradyarrhythmias.

Sinus arrest

When there is a failure of the SA node to generate an impulse, that is, the SA node has temporarily arrested – it is referred to as **sinus arrest.** Sinus arrest is commonly only a few to several seconds in duration, and when there is a prolonged pause, there is usually an escape beat (or escape rhythm). If sinus arrest exceeds 10–15 seconds without an escape rhythm (i.e. complete absence of cardiac contractions), then the blood pressure will fall and syncope will occur. If this does occur, there is usually a surge in catecholamines that triggers a return of a sinus rhythm or escape rhythm, which is typically fairly rapid.

ECG characteristics

There is a pause in the rhythm with neither a P wave nor, therefore, a QRS–T complex, that is, the baseline is flat (except for movement artefact if present) (Fig. 7.1). Long periods of arrest are often followed by ventricular escape complexes (Chapter 4).

Clinical findings

A pause in the heart rhythm will be heard on auscultation (with no palpable pulse); it will effectively sound as if the heart has briefly stopped. The duration of the pause (silence) will depend on the duration of the period of sinus arrest and if it is occurring episodically or not.

Sick sinus syndrome

This is a term for an abnormally functioning SA node in which it fails to trigger normal sinus complexes; it is, therefore, sometimes

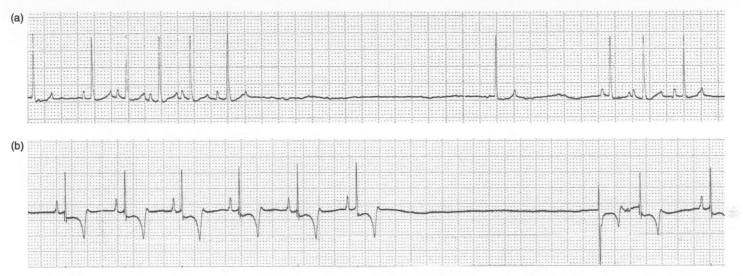

Figure 7.1 (a) ECG showing a short episode of sinus arrest lasting 3 seconds in an older West Highland White terrier with idiopathic pulmonary fibrosis (25 mm/s and 10 mm/mV). (b) ECG from a West Highland White terrier with sinus arrest, followed by a ventricular escape beat (25 mm/s and 10 mm/mV).

also termed **sinus node dysfunction**. Oftentimes, there is an absence of an escape rhythm, combined with a variety of bradyarrhythmias. This 'umbrella' term refers to any abnormality of sinus node function including sinus bradycardia and sinus arrest. Sometimes, when there is a junctional escape rhythm, there are preceding P waves with an abnormal morphology, typically negative. Sometimes, there are non-conducted P waves (see heart block later) intermingled with a variety of bradyarrhythmias. In some situations, the profound bradycardia alternates with a supraventricular tachycardia; this is termed the **'bradycardia–tachycardia syndrome'.** Sick sinus syndrome (SSS) has been reported to occur most commonly in female miniature Schnauzers

of at least 6 years of age and in West Highland White and Cairn terriers. It has not been recorded in cats.

ECG characteristics

The electrocardiographic features are, therefore, quite variable and include persistent sinus bradycardia or episodes of sinus arrest without escape beats. One feature of SSS is that during long periods of sinus arrest, there is often a failure of an escape rhythm to develop. In the bradycardia–tachycardia syndrome, there are periods of bradycardia such as sinus arrest, alternating with a supraventricular tachycardia

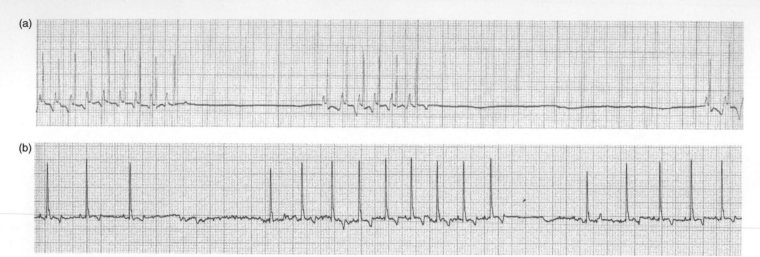

Figure 7.2 (a) ECG from a West Highland White terrier with alternating sinus arrest pauses with a sinus tachycardia; (b) ECG from a Cairn terrier with alternating sinus tachycardia with sinus arrest; these are alternating types of rhythms termed bradycardia–tachycardia sick sinus syndrome.

typically exceeding 200/min (Fig. 7.2). The bradycardia may be unresponsive to atropine.

Clinical findings

The findings on auscultation are very variable, from a markedly slow heart rate, to a variable rhythm, or with long pauses (associated with sinus arrest). The bradycardia–tachycardia syndrome sounds like periods of slow heart rate or pauses (silence), alternating with periods of very fast heart rate, and not necessarily with any regularity. There may be pulse deficits during the tachycardic episodes and no pulse produced during the periods of arrest.

Atrial standstill

In atrial standstill, there is an absence of atrial activity, that is, a continuous absence of P waves. Atrial standstill occurs due to a failure of atrial muscle depolarisation; that is, the SA node may produce an impulse but the atria are not depolarised and remain inactive. Most commonly in animals, this is associated with **hyperkalaemia** or **atrial cardiomyopathy**.

Hyperkalaemia (which often has a concurrent hyponatraemia) results in dysfunction of the action potential within the atrial myocytes, resulting in a failure of atrial depolarisation (also see hyperkalaemia in Chapter 8). This is progressive and starts with P waves that are smaller than normal, progressively reducing in size until there is complete

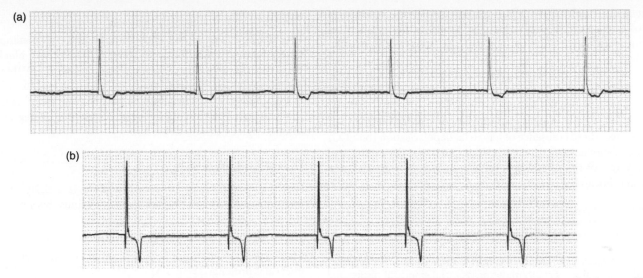

Figure 7.3 (a) ECG from a miniature Schnauzer and (b) a Border collie, both with atrial standstill with a nodal escape rhythm at 60/min. Note the absence of P waves. The absence of atrial activity can be confirmed by echocardiography (25 mm/s and 10 mm/mV). Fig. 7.3b courtesy of Jo Dukes McEwan.

absence with no P waves; that is atrial standstill. The impulses are conducted from the SA node by internodal pathways to the AV node, which is termed a **sinoventricular rhythm**.

Atrial cardiomyopathy is another cause of atrial standstill, usually affecting both atria and resulting in congestive heart failure. In this condition, the atrial myocytes fail to depolarise because they are diseased and so fail to contract.

Whether atrial standstill is associated with hyperkalaemia or atrial cardiomyopathy, the ECG tracing looks similar.

ECG characteristics

The main electrocardiographic feature is the absence of P waves, usually with a slow junctional or ventricular escape rhythm (usually less than 60/min) (Fig. 7.3). The quality of the ECG has to be excellent (i.e. the baseline must be flat without any artefacts) to diagnose the absence of P waves confidently. In search of very small P waves, an ECG can be recorded using precordial chest leads or using transthoracic leads. Additionally, the absence of atrial contractions and/or AV valve movement can be confirmed by echocardiography. The QRS complexes are often of a relatively normal shape (junctional escape), sometimes with a slightly prolonged duration, but there can also be a ventricular escape rhythm.

If animals with hyperkalaemia are presented early in the course of the disease, small P waves may be evident prior to atrial standstill. With hyperkalaemia, T waves often become taller as well.

Very rarely, in the cases of atrial cardiomyopathy in which only the left atrium is affected, there is absence of left atrial depolarisation (on ECG) and absence of movement (on echocardiography); yet the presence of very tiny P waves of right atrial depolarisation and of right atrial contractions (on echocardiography) – this can mimic complete heart block.

> **Note: Differentiation between sinus arrest and atrial standstill**
>
> Sinus arrest produces a 'flatline' that is *intermittent* (in between periods of a normal sinus rhythm), whereas atrial standstill results in a continuous absence of P waves while there is an underlying escape rhythm.

Clinical findings

The normal heart sounds will be heard (and associated pulse felt) in association with ventricular depolarisation. The rate will vary in each case, although generally it is slower than normal (often less than 60/min). Note: in comparison with heart block (see below), no atrial contraction sounds are heard.

> **Note:** While the clinical findings on examination of a patient are discussed here, the clinical significance of bradyarrhythmias is discussed in Chapter 15.

Heart block

This is the failure of the depolarisation wave to conduct normally through the AV node; the correct term is therefore AV block; however, heart block is often used as a synonymous term. AV block may be partial (first- or second-degree block) or complete (third-degree block). Advanced second-degree and complete heart block are usually associated with clinical signs, whereas first-degree and mild second-degree heart block are not.

First-degree AV block

First-degree AV block occurs when there is a delay in conduction through the AV node and there is usually a sinus rhythm.

ECG characteristics

The P wave and QRS complexes are normal in configuration, but the PR interval is prolonged (Fig. 7.4).

Clinical findings

No abnormality will be appreciated on auscultation or palpation of the pulse, and it cannot be distinguished from a normal sinus rhythm.

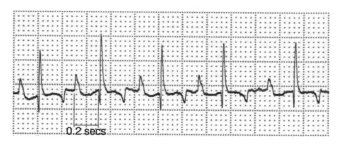

Figure 7.4 ECG from a miniature Schnauzer showing a prolonged P–R interval of 0.18 to 0.2 s, this is first-degree AV block (25 mm/s and 10 mm/mV).

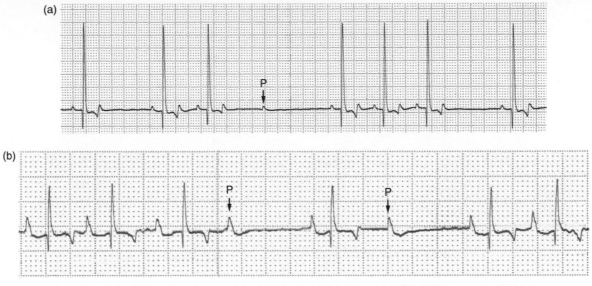

Figure 7.5 (a) ECG from a dog during anaesthesia showing a P-wave (arrowed) not followed by a QRS complex. (b) ECG from a miniature Schnauzer (same ECG as in Fig. 7.4), which also shows non-conducted P waves. These both are examples of second-degree AV block. (25 mm/s and 10 mm/mV).

Second-degree AV block

Second-degree AV block occurs when conduction intermittently fails to pass through the AV node that is, there is atrial depolarisation that is not followed by ventricular depolarisation. This is sometimes also referred to as a 'non-conducted' P wave.

ECG characteristics

The P wave is normal, but there is either an occasional or a frequent failure (depending on severity) of conduction through the AV node resulting in the absence of a QRS complex (Fig. 7.5).

Second-degree AV block can be classified further. When the P–R interval increases prior to the block, it is termed **Mobitz type I** (also known as **Wenckebach's phenomenon**). But when the P–R interval remains constant prior to the block, it is termed **Mobitz type II**, and the frequency of the block is usually constant, that is, 2:1, 3:1 and so on (Fig. 7.6).

Clinical findings

There will be occasional pauses in the rhythm associated with the absence of ventricular depolarisation. On very careful auscultation, the atrial contraction sounds (A-sounds or S4) can often be appreciated as a faint background noise (in association with atrial depolarisation).

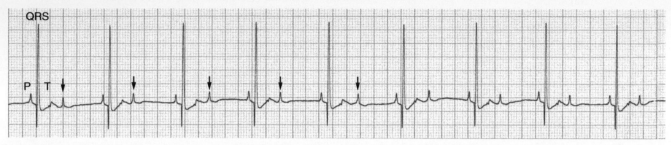

Figure 7.6 ECG from a Labrador, which shows alternating sinus complexes with non-conducted P waves (arrowed) (second-degree AV block). The 2:1 relationship is an example of Mobitz type II (25 mm/s and 10 mm/mV).

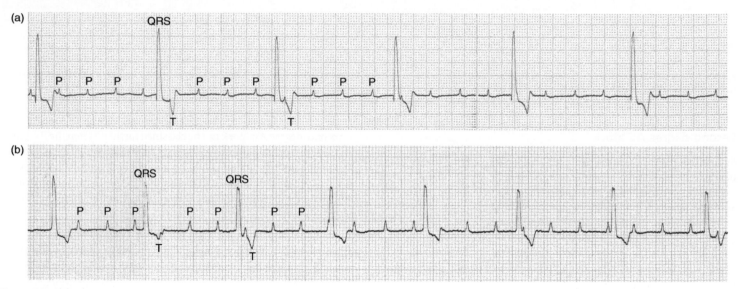

Figure 7.7 ECGs from a Lurcher (a) and a Wire Haired Fox terrier (b) with complete (third-degree) AV block with a nodal escape rhythm (both at 25 mm/s and 5 mm/mV).

60

Complete (third-degree) AV block

Complete AV block occurs when there is a persistent failure of the depolarisation wave to be conducted through the AV node. A second latent pacemaker below the AV node discharges to depolarise the ventricles. This second pacemaker may arise from:

- Lower AV node or bundle branches producing a normal QRS (i.e. junctional escape complex) at approximately 60–70/min (in dogs) (Fig. 7.7)

- Purkinje cells producing an abnormal QRS–T complex (i.e. ventricular escape complex) at approximately 30–40/min (in dogs) (Fig. 7.8)
- In cats, the escape rhythm can be either nodal or ventricular, or a mixture of both, often at a rate of 100–130/min.

ECG characteristics

On the ECG, P waves can be seen at a regular and fast rate, however, the QRS–T complexes are at a much slower rate and usually fairly regular. The P waves and QRS complexes occur independently of each other

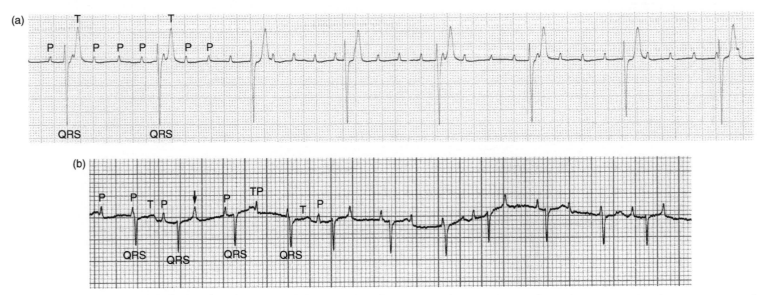

Figure 7.8 ECG from a Cocker Spaniel (a) and DSH cat (b) with complete (third-degree) AV block with a ventricular escape rhythm. There is an occasional P wave superimposed on a T wave, resulting in a summated deflection (arrowed) (25 mm/s and 10 mm/mV). Fig. 7.8b courtesy of Anne French.

(Figs 7.7 & 7.8). This is best demonstrated by plotting out each P wave and each QRS complex on a piece of paper.

Clinical findings

In many cases, the ventricular escape rhythm associated with complete heart block is very regular (often quite metronomic), although slow. So a regular slow bradycardia is heard with normally a good palpable pulse (sometimes, the escape rhythm is not regular). On very careful auscultation (sometimes using the bell of the stethoscope), the atrial contraction sounds (S4) can be faintly heard at a faster rate and not related to the normal lubb-dub of ventricular contraction.

Ventricular standstill

The absence of any ventricular activity is termed ventricular standstill. This results in the absence of ventricular contraction and, thus, an acute fall in blood pressure and, therefore, syncope. If there is no return of ventricular contractions, then sudden death will occur.

ECG characteristics

No ventricular rhythm is present.

This may occur with sinus arrest (see page 55) and the prolonged failure of an escape rhythm, or it may be seen with complete heart block (Fig. 7.9), with the absence of the ventricular escape rhythm; the P waves are usually seen to continue, but no ventricular rhythm is present. This is a common cause of syncope in dogs with complete heart block.

Clinical findings

No heart sounds will be heard, or pulse palpable, during the period of ventricular standstill. If this is associated with heart block, then faint atrial contractions may be heard, but if associated with sinus arrest, nothing will be heard.

Asystole

The sustained absence of any cardiac electrical activity (i.e., no P waves and no QRS complexes) is termed asystole. It is colloquially known as a 'flatline'. This leads to death, unless there is a return of electrical activity and cardiopulmonary resuscitation (CPR) should be initiated.

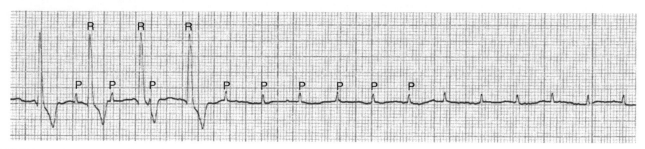

Figure 7.9 ECG from a Weimaraner with complete (third-degree) AV block, but additionally with episodes of ventricular standstill (which resulted in collapse) (25 mm/s and 10 mm/mV).

8 • Changes in the P–QRS–T morphology

Wandering pacemaker

This occurs as a result of the dominant pacemaker shifting from the SA node to other pacemaker cells with a high intrinsic rate within the atria. This is sometimes referred to as a wandering atrial pacemaker. This is a normal variant and not uncommon in dogs. It is thought to be associated with high vagal tone. Its significance is therefore similar to sinus arrhythmia (Chapter 3).

ECG characteristics

P waves can vary in morphology, that is, there is a variation in amplitude, varying from positive, negative or biphasic, or they can even be isoelectric (i.e. they can be so small that they are difficult to identify) (Fig. 8.1).

Changes associated with chamber enlargement

Prior to the advent of echocardiography, ECGs were originally used to aid in deciding if there was heart enlargement. However, the accuracy of ECGs for the assessment of heart enlargement is now known to be poor; therefore, screening for heart enlargement should no longer be the sole reason for performing electrocardiography.

Note that in 'ECG-speak', 'enlargement' is commonly used to encompass either hypertrophy or dilation, as these can rarely be distinguished reliably on an ECG.

Table 8.1 lists the normal values of ECG complex durations and amplitudes. Measurements are usually made in lead II at 50 mm/s, unfiltered.

Left atrial enlargement

When there is left atrial (LA) enlargement (or dilation), the P wave is often prolonged and sometimes also notched (Fig. 8.2). A prolonged and notched P wave is referred to as **P-mitrale** (as LA enlargement is often associated with mitral valve disease). The notching occurs as a result of asynchronous depolarisation of the atria, the dilated left atrium depolarising fractionally at a later stage as compared to the right atrium. Note: giant breeds often normally have slightly prolonged P waves.

Small Animal ECGs: An Introductory Guide, Third Edition. Mike Martin.
© 2015 John Wiley & Sons, Ltd. Published 2015 by John Wiley & Sons, Ltd.

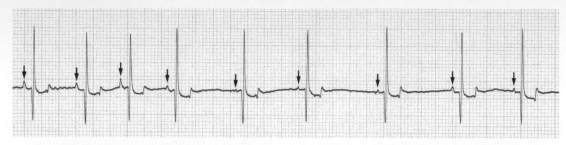

Figure 8.1 ECG from a dog showing a wandering pacemaker. Note how the P wave morphology changes (arrows) (lead II, 25 mm/s and 10 mm/mV).

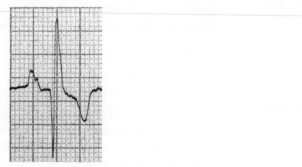

Figure 8.2 ECG illustrating prolonged (0.06 seconds) and notched P waves; this is termed P-mitrale. From a 10-year-old CKCS with mitral valve disease (50 mm/s and 10 mm/mV).

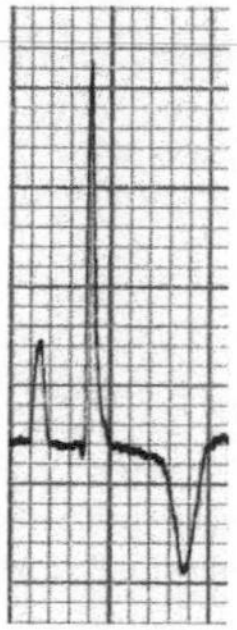

Figure 8.3 ECG illustrating tall P waves (0.5 mV); this is termed P-pulmonale. From a 10-year-old WHWT with idiopathic pulmonary fibrosis (25 mm/sec and 10 mm/mV).

Right atrial enlargement

When there is right atrial (RA) enlargement (or dilation), the P wave is increased in amplitude (Fig. 8.3). Such tall P waves are referred to as **P-pulmonale** (as RA enlargement may be associated with cor pulmonale). Note that P-pulmonale is commonly seen in breeds that are predisposed to chronic airway disease.

Left ventricular enlargement

Tall R waves are suggestive of left ventricular (LV) enlargement (Fig. 8.4). An R wave in lead I greater than that in lead II or aVF may be associated with hypertrophy. An increase in R waves in leads I, II and III maybe associated with dilation. Other ECG features that maybe associated with LV enlargement are: prolongation of the QRS duration, S–T segment sagging/coving and a shift in the mean electrical axis (MEA) to the left.

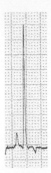

Figure 8.4 ECG illustrating tall R waves (4.0 mV), which is suggestive of left ventricular enlargement. From an 8-year-old CKCS with MVD (25 mm/s and 10 mm/mV).

Right ventricular enlargement

Deep S waves are suggestive of right ventricular (RV) enlargement (Fig. 8.5). Other ECG features that may be associated with RV enlargement are: prolongation of the QRS duration or a shift in the MEA to the right.

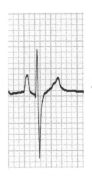

Figure 8.5 ECG illustrating deep S waves in lead II. From a 1-year-old miniature Dachshund with pulmonic stenosis (25 mm/s and 10 mm/mV).

Low-voltage QRS complexes

QRS complexes will be smaller the further the electrodes are from the heart and depend on the resistance to electrical conduction between the heart and the electrodes. For example, the ECG complexes are larger in precordial chest leads, which are very close to the heart. However, complexes can be small in the limb leads in obese animals. Heavy filtering on the ECG machine can also reduce the amplitude of the ECG complexes significantly.

Small complexes in dogs maybe associated with obesity, effusions (pericardial, pleural, ascites), hypothyroidism, hyperkalaemia, pneumothorax, some respiratory diseases, and hypovolaemia, or it may be a normal variation.

ECG characteristics

An R wave amplitude less than 0.5 mV in the limb leads is considered small in dogs (Fig. 8.6). QRS complexes are usually small in normal cats.

Electrical alternans

This is an alternation in QRS amplitude that occurs nearly every other beat (Fig. 8.7).

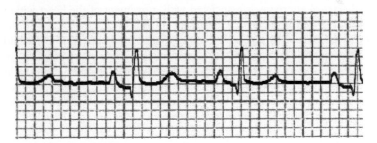

Figure 8.6 ECG illustrating small ECG complexes in a dog with pericardial effusion (25 mm/s and 10 mm/mV).

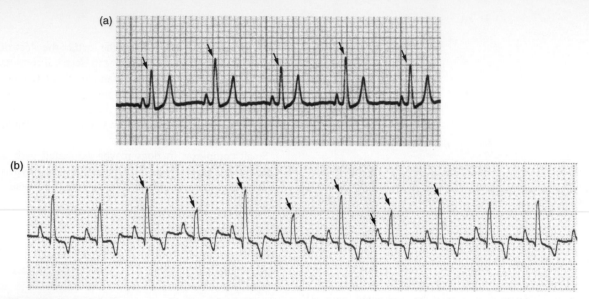

Figure 8.7 ECGs illustrating electrical alternans – note the alternating amplitude of the R waves. From a Golden Retriever (a) and a Greyhound (b) with pericardial effusion due to idiopathic pericarditis (25 mm/s and 10 mm/mV).

Electrical alternans is associated with movement of the heart within pericardial effusion, which is evident on echocardiography where the heart can be seen to 'bounce' from side to side within the pericardial fluid as it beats. This movement of the heart causes a slight alternating change in the cardiac axis and is seen on the ECG as an alternating variation in QRS amplitude. Note: this should not be confused with the more gradual variation in amplitude seen with respiration in some animals, nor the variation seen with a supraventricular tachycardia or atrial fibrillation.

Q–T interval abnormalities

The Q–T interval varies slightly, inversely with heart rate; so it is difficult to accurately define what is exactly abnormal.

Prolonged Q–T intervals (Fig. 8.8) may be seen in:

- hypocalcaemia
- hypokalaemia
- hypothermia

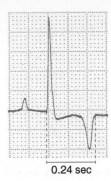

0.24 sec

Figure 8.8 ECG illustrating a prolonged QT interval in a dog (50 mm/s and 10 m/mV).

- quinidine
- ethylene glycol poisoning.

Shortened Q–T interval may be seen in:

- hyperkalaemia
- hypercalcaemia
- digitalis
- atropine
- β-blockers and calcium channel antagonists.

S–T segment abnormalities

S–T depression (Fig. 8.9) may be seen in:

- myocardial ischaemia (e.g. cardiomyopathy, trauma)
- potassium imbalance
- digitalis toxicity.

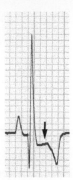

Figure 8.9 ECG illustrating depression of the S–T segment (arrowed). From a CKCS with mitral valve disease (25 mm/s and 10 mm/mV).

S–T elevation may be seen in:

- pericarditis (pericardial effusion)
- severe ischaemia/infarction, e.g. full wall thickness.

Abnormalities of the T wave

The morphology of T waves in small animals is very variable and the diagnostic value of T wave changes is very limited when compared with that in humans. A higher value might be placed on the T wave changes compared with a previous recording in the same animal. The most common abnormal change is the development of larger peaked T waves; this can be associated with hyperkalaemia (see below) or myocardial hypoxia.

Hyperkalaemia

Hyperkalaemia is a well-known cause of ECG abnormalities (Fig. 8.10), however, it must be remembered that a normal ECG would not exclude

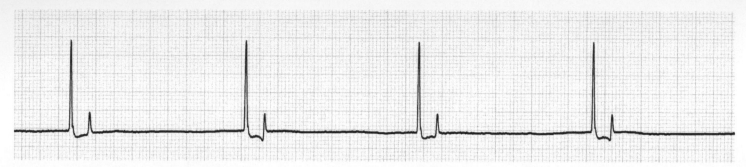

Figure 8.10 ECG illustrating a bradycardia at 30/min, the absence of P waves (atrial standstill) and slightly peaked T waves from a dog with hyperkalaemia (25 mm/s and 10 mm/mV). ECG tracing courtesy of Paul Wotton.

hyperkalaemia (e.g. Addison's disease), and serum electrolyte levels should always be measured (and an adrenocorticotropic hormone test performed) if this is suspected.

Hyperkalaemia may be associated with Addison's disease, acute renal shutdown (e.g. feline urethral obstruction syndrome), diabetic ketoacidosis and severe skeletal muscle damage.

ECG characteristics

The ECG changes vary with increasing severity of the hyperkalaemia as follows:

- there is a progressive bradycardia
- increased amplitude of the T wave, appearing narrow and spiked
- progressive decrease in amplitude of the R wave
- progressive reduction in amplitude of the P wave
- disappearance of the P wave, i.e. atrial standstill (see page 56), with a slow junctional (nodal) rhythm
- finally, ventricular fibrillation or asystole.

Note: The presence or severity of hyperkalaemia does not reliably correlate with the changes in the ECG tracing; serum levels must be measured if hyperkalaemia is ever suspected.

Table 8.1 Guidelines on normal values for cats and dogs when ECG is recorded in right lateral recumbency.

		Dog	Cat
Heart rate	Adult	70–160	120–240
	Puppy	70–220	
Measurements			
P wave duration		<0.04 s	<0.04 s
	Giant breeds	<0.05 s	
P wave amplitude		<0.4 mV	<0.2 mV
P–R interval		0.06–0.13 s	0.05–0.09 s
QRS duration		<0.05 s	<0.04 s
	Giant breeds	<0.06 s	
R wave amplitudes		<2.0 mV	<0.9 mV
	Giant breeds	<2.5 mV	
S–T segment	Depression	<0.2 mV	No depression
	Elevation	<0.15 mV	No elevation
T wave		<0.25 of normal R wave amplitude	<0.3 MV
Q–T interval		0.15–0.25 s	0.12–0.18 s
Mean electrical axis		+40° to +100°	0° to + 160°

Source: L. P. Tilley (1992) *Essentials of Canine and Feline Electrocardiography: Interpretation and Treatment*, 3rd edn, Lea & Febiger.

PART 3
More advanced electrocardiography

An understanding of the ECG lead systems is necessary to understand both the cardiac electrical axis (Chapter 10) and intraventricular conduction defects (Chapter 11).

The six ECG limb leads

In Chapters 2 and 3, the +ve and −ve electrodes, as shown in the diagrams, were placed so as to obtain a recording of the electricity of the heart. This *combination* of a +ve and a −ve electrode is termed a **bipolar lead**, simply meaning between two poles, that is, a +ve and a −ve pole (electrodes). For example, lead 2 is formed by the right foreleg electrode being the negative pole and the left hind leg electrode being the positive pole. Leads 1, 2 and 3 are all bipolar leads (Fig. 9.1a–c). However, the term 'lead' can cause confusion, as an ECG cable or wire is often also called an ECG 'lead' in ECG-speak. This potential confusion should be avoided.

While there are usually four ECG electrodes, one of these is an earth (the electrode on the right hind leg). The other three are the active electrodes to which the −ve and +ve terminals are connected. All ECG electrodes are labelled and/or colour coded for identification (Table 9.1), to ensure correct placement on each of the limbs (although the colour codings in Europe and in America are not the same).

Table 9.1 ECG cable colour coding.

Limb	International	American	Labelling often on human electrodes
Right fore	Red	White	RA (right arm)
Left fore	Yellow	Black	LA (left arm)
Left hind	Green	Red	LL (left leg)
Right hind (earth)	Black	Green	RL (right leg)

When the ECG electrodes are attached to the animal, switching the 'channels' on the ECG machine can provide different bipolar leads as shown in Fig. 9.1. It can be seen how three ECG electrodes can provide a total combination of six ECG bipolar leads.[1] Thus the six limb bipolar leads 'look at' the heart in six different directions.

[1] A small portion of 'poetic license' is used in this statement. Correctly, leads 1, 2 and 3 are bipolar leads; however, leads aVR, aVL and aVF are augmented unipolar leads. Unipolar leads measure the electrical potential between a positive electrode and a central terminal created electronically within the circuitry of the ECG machine by combining the electric currents obtained from the other two electrodes. The deflections are smaller than those of the bipolar leads, and thus they are also augmented (1.5 times).

Small Animal ECGs: An Introductory Guide, Third Edition. Mike Martin.
© 2015 John Wiley & Sons, Ltd. Published 2015 by John Wiley & Sons, Ltd.

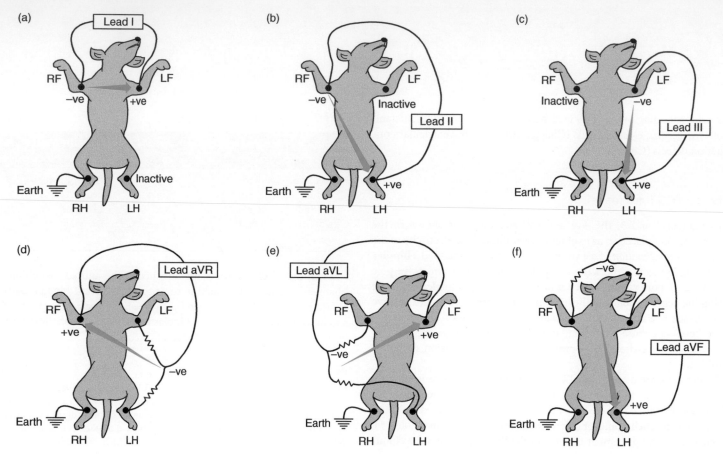

Figure 9.1 These diagrams illustrate how the six limb leads are generated by switching the electrode connections. The RH electrode is always the earth and does not form part of the bipolar electrode. (a) When the ECG machine is switched to select lead 1 – the RF becomes the −ve electrode and the LF the +ve electrode. (b) When lead 2 is selected, the RF becomes the −ve electrode and the LH the +ve electrode. (c) When lead 3 is selected, the LF becomes the −ve electrode and the LH the +ve electrode. (d) When lead aVR is selected, a combination of the LF and LH becomes the −ve electrode, and the RF becomes the +ve electrode. (e) When lead aVL is selected, the −ve electrode is the combination of the RF and LH, and the +ve electrode is the LF. (f) When lead aVF is selected, the −ve electrode is the combination of the RF and LF, and the +ve electrode is the LH. The 'blue-coloured' arrows show the direction of each of the leads viewing the depolarisation wave as it travels through the heart.

10 • Mean electrical axis (MEA) explained

The mean electrical axis (MEA), also referred to as the cardiac axis, is rarely used in veterinary cardiology. So, you might ask, why is it being explained in this book? Well, an understanding of the MEA develops a better understanding of the 'electricity of the heart' and, therefore, of the interpretation of ECG tracings. Additionally, an understanding of the MEA greatly helps in the understanding of intraventricular conduction blocks in the next chapter.

Understanding the mean electrical axis (MEA)

Although depolarisation waves spread through the heart in 'all directions', the average direction and magnitude is represented by the QRS complex. If the QRS is predominantly positive (upwards), the average direction of the depolarisation waves is toward the +ve electrode. Conversely, if it is predominantly negative (downwards), then the depolarisation wave is moving away from the +ve electrode. When the QRS complex is equally positive and negative (and usually small), then the depolarisation wave might be moving at right angles to the +ve electrode.

The limb leads 'look at' the heart from six different directions (Fig. 9.1). The average direction and magnitude of the depolarisation wave through the ventricles are together termed the **mean electrical axis (MEA)** or the

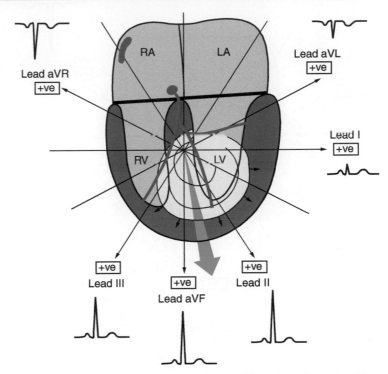

Figure 10.1 The normal mean electrical axis (large 'blue-coloured' arrow) and how this is 'seen' from each of the six limb leads. Note that leads 2 and aVF, in this example, produce ECG tracings with the tallest (most positive) QRS complexes – this is often the case in the vast majority of dogs and cats with a normal heart. This is also the reason why we mostly perform an ECG rhythm strip on lead 2. RA – right atrium; LA – left atrium; RV – right ventricle; LV – left ventricle.

Small Animal ECGs: An Introductory Guide, Third Edition. Mike Martin.
© 2015 John Wiley & Sons, Ltd. Published 2015 by John Wiley & Sons, Ltd.

cardiac axis. As can be seen from Fig. 10.1, in which there is a normal axis, leads I, II, III and aVF have positive deflections, and aVR and aVL are negative.

Right axis deviation

If the right ventricle becomes enlarged as illustrated (Fig. 10.2) (through either hypertrophy or dilation), then the MEA swings to the right, because the large increase in muscle mass on the right side creates a larger electrical potential difference during depolarisation.

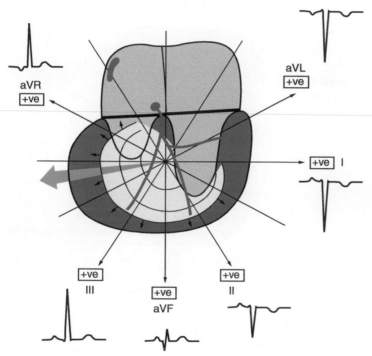

Figure 10.2 The mean electrical axis (large 'blue-coloured' arrow) in an animal with right ventricular enlargement (RVE) and how this is 'seen' from the six limb leads. Note how lead 3 now becomes more positive, as compared to lead 2 (for example), and also how aVR (which usually has a negative QRS complex) has now become positive. This is termed a right axis shift. Conditions associated with right ventricular enlargement can produce a right axis shift, such as pulmonic stenosis, tricuspid dysplasia or cor pulmonale.

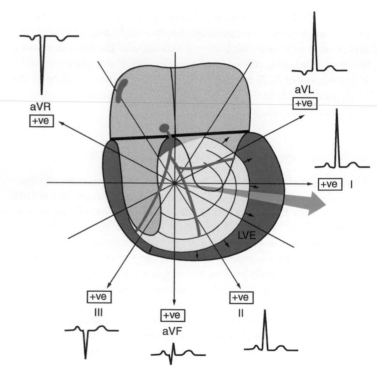

Figure 10.3 The mean electrical axis (large 'blue-coloured' arrow) in an animal with left ventricular enlargement (LVE) and how this is 'seen' from the six limb leads. Note how leads 1 and aVL now become more positive, as compared to lead 3 (for example). This is termed a left axis shift. Conditions associated with left ventricular enlargement can produce a right axis shift, such as a PDA, MVD or DCM.

As shown in Fig. 10.2, for example, leads III and aVR become large and positive. Leads I, II and aVL become negative. Lead aVF is isoelectric in this example. This is termed a right axis deviation.

Left axis deviation

If the left ventricle becomes enlarged (through either hypertrophy or dilation), then the MEA swings to the left, because the large increase in muscle mass on the left side creates a large electrical potential difference during depolarisation.

As shown in Fig. 10.3, for example, lead I becomes taller than lead II. Lead aVL is also positive. Leads III and aVR are negative, and aVF is isoelectric. This is termed a left axis deviation.

How to calculate the mean electrical axis

This is of limited value in small animals, in part because the vector in the frontal plane (which is the plane that is measured from the limb leads) is less representative of the true direction of the vector in three dimensions, as compared with humans. The MEA is used mainly to assist in the assessment of ventricular enlargement and in the recognition of intraventricular conduction defects.

The value obtained in exactly measuring the MEA in every case is questionable; a rough estimate of whether it is right or left is usually sufficient. However, the understanding of how it is measured and how it varies provides a deeper understanding of the 'electricity of the heart'.

How to estimate the MEA

There are a few methods of measuring the MEA; two are described here.

Eyeballing the MEA

Using this method provides a quick system and, with practice, the MEA can often be 'eyeballed' to see whether it is normal or abnormal. Look

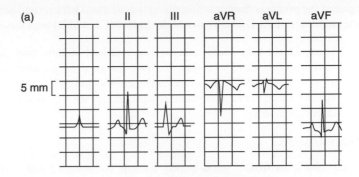

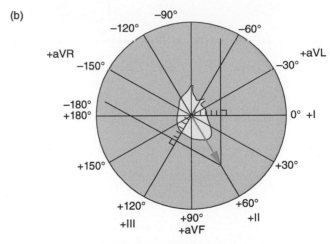

Figure 10.4 Estimation of mean electrical axis. (a) *Method 1*. In this normal canine ECG, lead aVL is the most isoelectric lead. Perpendicular to this is lead II. Lead II is positive, and therefore the MEA is towards the positive pole of this line, that is, +60°. (b) *Method 2*. In the same ECG, the net amplitude in lead I is +6 (Q = 0 and R = +6). Plot 6 points along lead I in the hexaxial lead system diagram and draw a perpendicular. The net amplitude in lead III is +6 (S = −2 and R = +8). Plot 6 points along lead III and draw a perpendicular. Draw an arrow from the centre to where the two perpendicular lines intersect. This is the direction of the MEA, that is, +60°.

again at the previous diagrams describing the right and left axes and how the amplitude of the QRS complex varies in leads I, II and III with these.

(i) Using all six limb leads and the hexaxial lead system, find the lead in which the QRS complexes have the greatest (positive) net amplitude – the MEA is approximately in this direction.
(ii) Similarly, find the most negative complexes; the MEA is opposite in direction to this.

Triangulation

Using two leads from a good-quality tracing, commonly leads I and III are used to measure the net amplitude of the QRS complex in each lead. In other words, measure the amplitude of the QRS complex that is positive and the amplitude that is negative. Subtract one (the smaller) from the other – this is the net amplitude. Plot this, to scale, on the hexaxial lead system as shown in Fig. 10.4. Draw perpendicular lines from each point. Where the two lines meet is the direction of the MEA from the centre point.

In fact, if the net amplitude in all six leads is calculated and plotted on the hexaxial lead system, the lines that are drawn perpendicular from each point *should* all meet at approximately the same point.

11 • Intraventricular conduction defects

Anatomy of the bundle branches

Having understood the ECG leads and mean electrical axis, we can now explain the abnormalities due to intraventricular conduction defects (also known as ventricular aberrancy).

The bundle of His divides into left and right bundle branches, supplying the left and right ventricles, respectively (Chapter 2, figure 2.1). The left bundle branch further divides into anterior and posterior fascicles. As well as conduction block occurring in the AV node (i.e. heart block), a conduction block can also occur in the bundle branches. The most commonly seen conduction defects in dogs are:

- Right bundle branch block (RBBB)
- Left bundle branch block (LBBB)

and in cats are:

- Left anterior fascicular block (LAFB).

These result in abnormal depolarisation patterns as there will be a delay in depolarisation of the part of the ventricles supplied by the affected conduction tissue. This is also referred to as **aberrant ventricular conduction** or **ventricular aberrancy**.

Right bundle branch block

RBBB occurs due to failure/delay of impulse conduction through the RBB. Depolarisation of the left ventricle occurs normally, but depolarisation of the right ventricular mass occurs through the myocardial cell tissue resulting in a very prolonged complex.

ECG characteristics

The QRS duration is prolonged (>0.07 s). The QRS complex has deep and usually slurred S waves in leads I, II, III and aVF and is positive in aVR and aVL. The MEA is to the right (Fig. 11.1). Note that RBBB needs to be differentiated from a right ventricular enlargement pattern.

Clinical findings

On auscultation, the heart sounds and rhythm will be normal with associated palpable pulses. In some dogs, with very careful auscultation, a split-second heart sound (S2) maybe heard, due to delayed closure of the pulmonic valve.

Small Animal ECGs: An Introductory Guide, Third Edition. Mike Martin.
© 2015 John Wiley & Sons, Ltd. Published 2015 by John Wiley & Sons, Ltd.

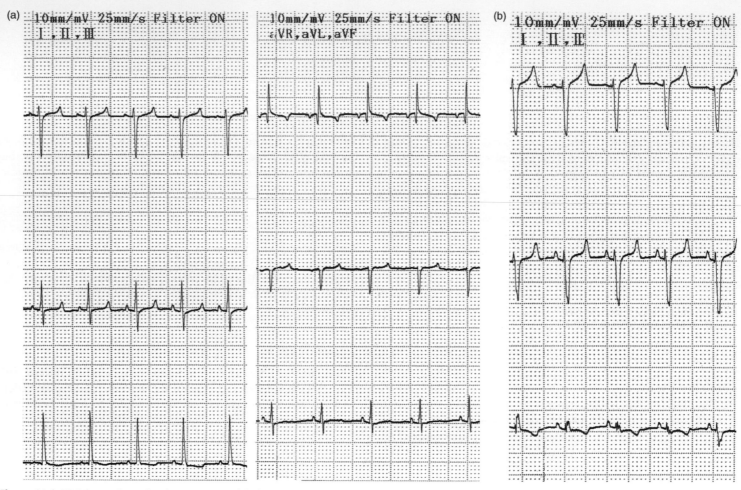

Figure 11.1 ECG from a dog with pulmonic stenosis. (a) This tracing shows all six limb leads, with a right axis deviation. (b) Following balloon dilation of the stenosis, RBBB develops. Note the change in QRS morphology to become prolonged in all 3 limb leads and inversion of the QRS in lead 2 as compared to pre-ballooning (25 mm/sec and 10 mm/mV).

Left bundle branch block

LBBB occurs due to failure of conduction through the LBB. Depolarisation of the right ventricle occurs normally, whereas depolarisation of the left ventricle is delayed and occurs through the myocardial cell tissue resulting in a very prolonged complex.

ECG characteristics

The QRS duration is very prolonged (>0.07 s). There are positive complexes in leads I, II, III and aVF and negative in aVR and aVL (Fig. 11.2). LBBB needs to be differentiated from a left ventricular enlargement pattern.

Clinical findings

The heart sounds and rhythm will sound normal with associated palpable pulses.

Left anterior fascicular block

LAFB occurs due to failure of conduction through the anterior fascicle of the LBB. It is not an uncommon finding in cats but is rare in dogs.

ECG characteristics

The QRS complex is normal in duration, but there are tall R waves in leads I and aVL, and deep S waves (>R wave) in leads II, III and aVF. The MEA is markedly to the left; approximately −60° in cats (Fig. 11.3).

Clinical findings

The heart sounds and rhythm will sound normal with associated palpable pulses.

More terminology to describe the morphology of VPCs

In Chapters 4 and 5, the morphology of VPCs was described as having a −ve or +ve QRS complex. In ECG-speak, however, the morphology of the QRS complex is described as being the same as LBBB or RBBB morphology. It is not until ventricular aberrancy has been explained that this terminology can be used.

In Boxer dogs with arrhythmogenic right ventricular cardiomyopathy, where the VPCs arise from the right ventricular outflow tract, they are described as VPCs with LBBB morphology.

Broad QRS complex tachycardia

This descriptive terminology was mentioned in Chapter 5 to describe a ventricular tachycardia (VT). If a dog with ventricular aberrancy (due to either RBBB or LBBB, as described earlier) then develops an SVT, then the rhythm will also look like a broad QRS complex tachycardia. In fact, one of the main reasons for using this descriptive terminology is because it can be very difficult to distinguish between an SVT with ventricular aberrancy and a VT. It is only when there is an interruption of the rhythm that hidden P waves might be seen (which would rule out a VT).

A very fast sinus tachycardia with ventricular aberrancy (in which the P waves cannot be clearly seen) can also be described as a broad QRS complex tachycardia and, therefore, mimic a VT.

A broad QRS complex tachycardia can be described as having an RBBB (Fig. 11.4a) or LBBB (Fig. 11.4b) morphology. The potential explanations for a broad QRS complex tachycardia are: VT, SVT with aberrancy and sinus tachycardia with aberrancy.

The combination of ventricular aberrancy with atrial fibrillation (AF) is also seen in dogs. One of the distinguishing features of this, as mentioned earlier, is the irregular rhythm caused by AF (and potentially the fibrillation waves).

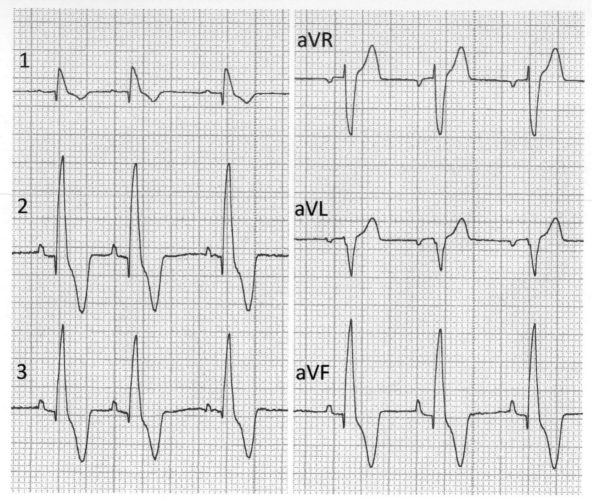

Figure 11.2 ECG from a Boxer dog with a normal sinus rhythm conducted through the ventricles with aberrancy due to left bundle branch block. Note the abnormal morphology of the QRS complexes, yet related to the P waves; that is, there is a P for every QRS, indicating the sinus origin of the depolarisation (25 mm/s and 10 mm/mV).

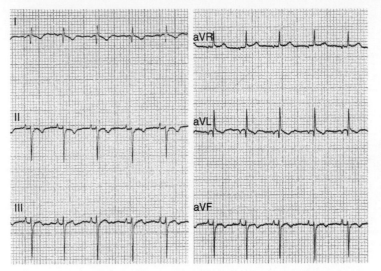

Figure 11.3 ECG from an 11year-old DSH cat with restrictive cardiomyopathy. There is a normal sinus rhythm but with aberrant ventricular conduction due to anterior fascicular block (see text) (25 mm/s and 10 mm/mV). ECG tracing courtesy of Dr Paul Wotton.

Ashman's phenomenon

This is a form of intermittent ventricular aberrancy due to a functional block.

When there is a longer than normal R–R interval, the refractory period also becomes longer. If there is a supraventricular premature that follows the long R–R interval, the premature depolarisation wave can encounter refractory tissue, resulting in aberrant ventricular conduction. It is most common to see RBBB morphology with Ashman's phenomenon as it is the right bundle that is usually slower to repolarise. This is a functional block, as opposed to a true (complete) bundle branch block.

Ashman's phenomenon can be seen in any cardiac rhythm when aberrant ventricular conduction occurs following a long ventricular cycle (R–R interval). More usually, it is seen with both supraventricular premature complexes and AF. As a consequence of Ashman's phenomenon, the abnormal broad QRS complex morphology and the premature timing can be misinterpreted as a VPC (Fig. 11.5) or potentially a paroxysm of VT.

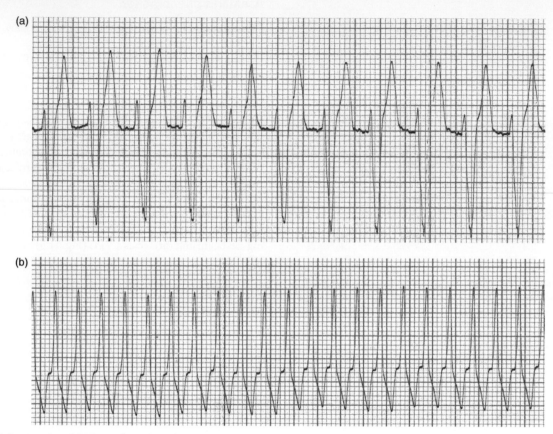

Figure 11.4 (a) ECG showing a broad QRS complex tachycardia with RBBB morphology. This can be due to either an SVT with ventricular aberrancy or a VT. (b) ECG showing a broad QRS complex tachycardia with LBBB morphology. This can be due to either an SVT with ventricular aberrancy or a VT.

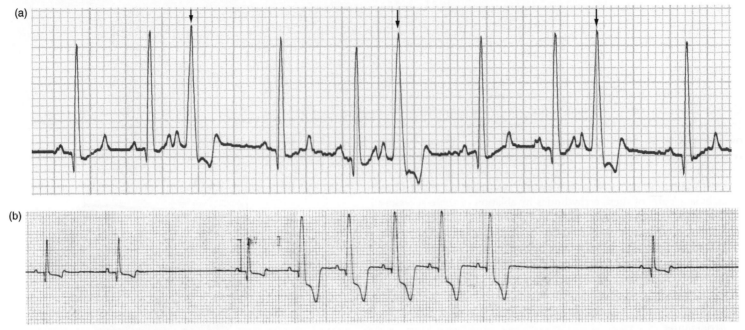

Figure 11.5 (a) ECG from a Gordon Setter. There is an underlying sinus rhythm with atrial premature complexes (APCs) (arrowed) with ventricular aberrancy initiated by Ashman's phenomenon. (b) ECG from a Labrador dog with a sinus rhythm. The first two sinus collapses are at a slow rate, which are then followed by a quicker sinus rhythm but with ventricular aberrancy; that is, the QRS morphology is indicative of left bundle branch block. In both of these examples, note how the QRS and T morphology associated with the quicker beats is different from the normal QRS and T; this is due to functional block (Ashman's phenomenon). Fig. 11.5b courtesy of Simon Dennis.

12 • Supraventricular arrhythmias: in-depth

Supraventricular arrhythmias in dogs: in-depth

Supraventricular arrhythmias were introduced and explained in Chapter 4 as 'any ectopic stimuli arising above the ventricles', which could arise from atrial tissue or the AV node. However, this was an over-simplification for teaching purposes. There are, in fact, several types of supraventricular arrhythmias based on their mechanism of action. Importantly, one of these arrhythmias is associated with accessory pathways (also known as bypass tracts). Treatment has now evolved to include a 'cure' of these arrhythmias by ablation of these accessory pathways, so this has now become an important topic to be explained.

Nearly all of this type of research has been conducted in dogs; hence this chapter only concerns dogs. Little is known about cats.

The three most common and important supraventricular arrhythmias in dogs are:

- Atrioventricular (AV) reciprocating tachycardia
- Focal atrial tachycardia (FAT)
- Atrial flutter

Note

Differentiating the different SVTs from the normal limb ECGs is very difficult, usually requiring an intracardiac electrophysiological study. But it is more important to be aware that SVTs are more complex than they might seem and expert advice should be sought, bearing in mind that there is the potential for ablation of the accessory pathway with good outcomes.

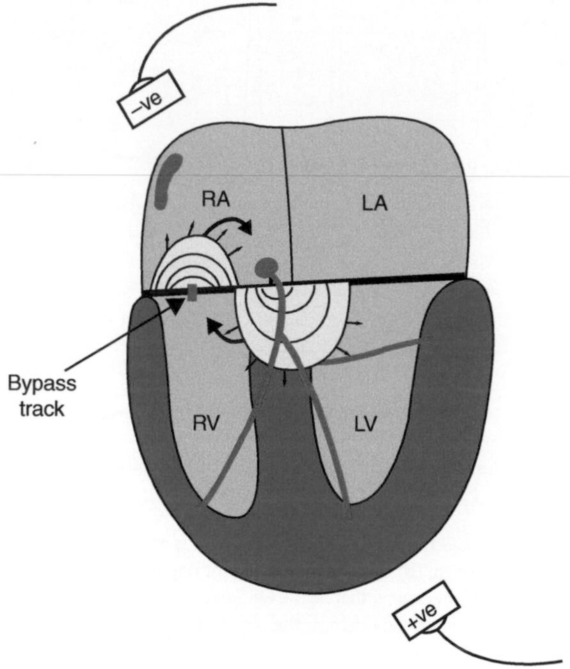

Figure 12.1 Diagram showing the electrical circuit in orthodromic atrioventricular reciprocating tachycardia (OAVRT). Conductions travels back up from the ventricles via a bypass tract to the atria, then back down the AV node, which develops a persistent re-entry circuit.

Atrioventricular reciprocating tachycardia

This arrhythmia is associated with congenital **AV accessory pathways**, which are muscular tracts connecting the atria and the ventricles, and thus bypassing the AV node. The accessory pathways are usually **concealed,** and what triggers the activation of these **bypass tracts** is not determined; however, when active, conduction of the electrical depolarisation wave occurs between the atria and the ventricles, and this can occur in either direction. This can therefore set up a circus movement tachycardia, also known as a **macro-reentrant tachycardia (Fig.** 12.1).

In dogs, the most common of these is **orthodromic atrioventricular reciprocating tachycardia(OAVRT):** when the electrical depolarisation wave travels down the AV node (in the normal, or orthodox, direction), depolarisation of the ventricles occurs, and when the depolarisation wave reaches the bypass tract, it is then conducted retrograde back up to the atria (Fig. 12.2). Depolarisation then travels back down the AV

node to the ventricles again and back up the bypass tract, completing the circuit. This has the potential to then set up a sustained rapid tachycardia. In contrast to FAT (described as follows), there is always a 1:1 atrioventricular conduction in dogs with OAVRT. Dogs can present with recurrent paroxysms of this SVT with episodic weakness, or present with a sustained SVT leading to tachycardia-induced myocardial failure and thus congestive heart failure signs. The most common breeds affected seem to be Labradors and Boxers and usually as young adult dogs. Cats with SVT can present with 'seizure-like' episodes.

ECG characteristics

- OAVRT is usually initiated during sinus rhythm but can also be initiated by an atrial or ventricular premature beat.
- The SVT starts and terminates abruptly, without 'warming up' or 'cooling down'.
- Termination by a VPC or APC is suggestive of OAVRT.

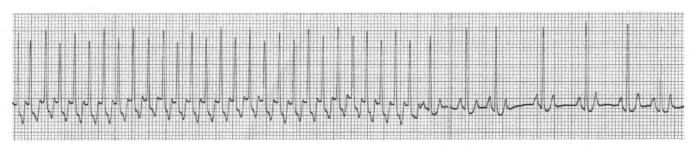

Figure 12.2 ECG from a Labrador that had a history of episodic weakness associated with rapid periods of SVT. In this tracing, the cessation of a long run of SVT at 360/min is seen following i/v injection with lidocaine (25 mm/s and 10 mm/mV).

- The heart rate during a period of SVT is often 300–400/min (in dogs), but can be less than 300/min.
- The R–R interval is typically very regular during a period of SVT (because there is a fixed or constant circuit).
- There is a 1:1 atrioventricular conduction, but because the rate is very fast, the P' is often hidden.
- A hidden P' negative wave (in lead 2) may be seen after the QRS complexes (best seen after the last QRS of a period of SVT); this is usually a positive P' wave in lead aVR.
- The duration of the RP interval (from the QRS complex to the following P' wave) is usually shorter than the PR interval, that is the ratio RP: PR < 1.0 (in contrast to FAT).
- During periods of sinus rhythm, pre-excitation may be seen, and this would be diagnostic of the presence of an accessory pathway.
- Electrical alternans is common (see also Chapter 8,), where there is a variation in the amplitude of the QRS complex.

Clinical findings

The SVT may be heard to suddenly start or stop, with a more normal rhythm in between.

During a period of SVT, the heart rate is typically very fast and regular, and the pulse will be weak.

> **Note**
>
> During a fast SVT (of any mechanism), sometimes there is a pulsus alternans; thus, only half the heart beats and pulses are heard or felt. Therefore, the 'apparent' heart rate can be half the true rate and potentially mislead the clinician into assuming that there is not a tachycardia. Whenever an SVT is suspected, an ECG recording should be performed.

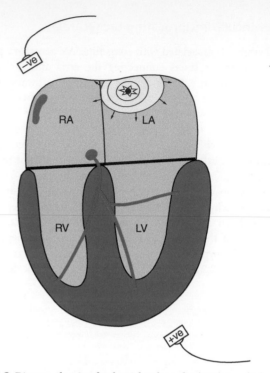

Figure 12.3 Diagram showing focal atrial tachycardia (FAT), in which a fast and repetitive ectopic focus within the atria generates a supraventricular tachycardia.

Focal atrial tachycardia

FAT is a rhythmic atrial focus that activates atrial depolarisation (and, consequently, ventricular depolarisation). The mechanism of action is thought to be due to abnormal automaticity or micro reentry (an explanation of these mechanisms is beyond the scope of this book). A sustained FAT can lead to tachycardia-induced myocardial failure in some dogs. FAT can also trigger the onset of atrial fibrillation (Fig. 12.3).

ECG characteristics

- The heart rate in dogs with FAT during SVT is typically 160–300/min (Fig. 12.4).
- At onset, usually an FAT starts relatively slower and then speeds up (warms up).
- At termination, it often seems to slow down a little before it stops (cools down).
- During a period of SVT, there is a narrow QRS complex morphology.
- The R–R interval can sometimes vary slightly, particularly with the warm-up and cool-down.
- The P–P interval often varies slightly (in contrast to atrial flutter).
- A hidden P′ positive wave (in lead 2) may be seen before the QRS complexes; this is often a negative P′ wave in lead aVR.
- The duration of the RP′ interval (from the QRS complex to the following P′ wave) is usually longer than the P′R interval, that is, the ratio RP′: P′R > 1.0 (in contrast to OAVRT).
- AV block occurs in one-third of dogs with this type of tachyarrhythmia, often with a 2:1 block, that is, 2 P′ waves to 1 QRS-T. The P′ waves are often hidden within the QRS-T complex, and thus the presence of AV block may not be seen. However, the AV block can be variable and produce a change in rates that would be characteristic.

Clinical findings

The SVT may be heard to suddenly start or stop, with a more normal rhythm in between.

During a period of SVT, the heart rate is typically very fast and usually regular with a weak pulse. Sometimes, there is a subtle and intermittent irregularity.

Atrial flutter

This is an uncommon arrhythmia in dogs. The arrhythmia is caused by a macro-reentry circuit within the right atrium. During atrial flutter, the atria discharge regularly at a rate of 250–400/min and conduction will travel down the AV node to depolarise the ventricles. Often there is AV block, which can be variable, that is, 2:1 or 3:1, for example. The rhythm can be regular, when there is a constant rate of AV conduction, that is,

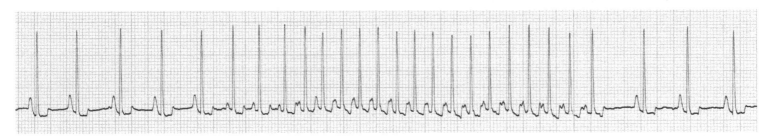

Figure 12.4 ECG from a Labrador with a history of episodic weakness. This dog was having very long runs of sustained SVT; however, this section of tracing shows a short paroxysm of SVT. Note that at the start of the SVT, there is a warm-up and at the end, a cool-down. The maximum heart rate during the SVT is 260/min here (25 mm/s and 10 mm/mV).

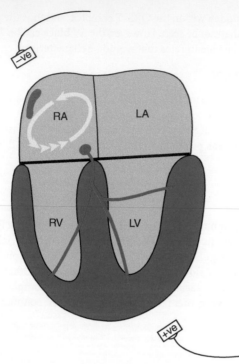

Figure 12.5 Diagram showing the electrical circuit associated with atrial flutter, in which there is a persistent re-entry pathway (in a section of the right atrium) resulting in a fast and persistent supraventricular tachycardia.

constantly 1:1 or constantly 2:1;but AV nodal conduction can also vary, creating an irregular rhythm that might mimic atrial fibrillation. If the flutter waves are seen (during a pause in the ventricular activity), they most commonly have a regular 'saw toothed' appearance, referred to as **typical atrial flutter**. In rare cases, the flutter can mimic very fast P waves, referred to as **atypical atrial flutter (Fig.** 12.5).

ECG characteristics

- Typical atrial flutter: the flutter waves (F waves) produce regular 'saw-toothed' deflections typically at a rate of 300–400/min, if seen (Fig. 12.6).
- Atypical atrial flutter: the P-like waves have a regular P–P interval (in contrast to FAT), typically at a rate of 300–400/min.
- During a period of SVT, there is a narrow QRS complex morphology.
- At high rates, there may be a functional AV block, thus producing a 2:1 or 3:1 conduction ratio.
- If the ventricular response rate is regular, the heart rate will also be regular; however, often, the conduction can be variable, producing an irregular heart rate (similar to atrial fibrillation).
- The R–R interval can be variable as the AV nodal conduction varies markedly.

Clinical findings

The heart rate is typically very fast and can be regular or irregular.

Note

Key message: If you got this far, you will appreciate that these SVTs are difficult to differentiate. The important point is to be aware that accessory pathways can be ablated (therefore, 'curing' the SVT); so do seek expert advice in the cases of SVT.

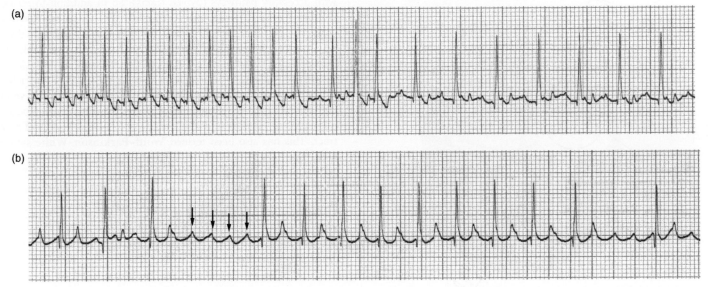

Figure 12.6 ECGs from a young Boxer dog, which presented with congestive heart failure secondary to a sustained SVT (i.e. tachycardia induced myocardial failure). (a) The tracings show an initial rapid heart rate of 300/min, which then reduces to 150/min. Initially, there is 1:1 conduction of the atrial flutter and then 2:1 conduction. (b) This section of tracing shows a long period of AV block, thus revealing the underlying flutter waves (arrowed) (25 mm/s and 10 mm/mV).

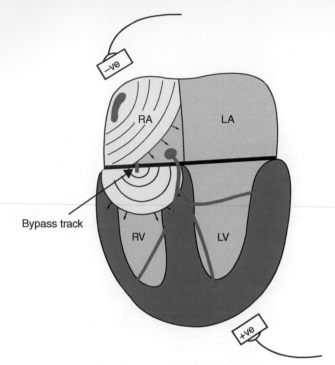

Figure 12.7 Diagram showing how pre-excitation of the ventricles occurs via conduction down a bypass tract.

Ventricular pre-excitation

Conduction of the electrical depolarisation wave can be bi-directional with accessory pathways (bypass tracts). So in addition to retrograde conduction up the bypass tract to trigger OAVRT, there can also be antegrade conduction down the bypass tract. In this instance, the depolarisation wave through the atria travels down the bypass tract to depolarise the ventricles before depolarisation of the AV node can depolarise the ventricles. This results in premature depolarisation of the ventricles: this is termed **ventricular pre-excitation**. In dogs with OAVRT, ventricular pre-excitation is seen in approximately one-third , during periods of normal sinus rhythm, and its presence would be indicative of a bypass tract. This has also been termed **Wolff–Parkinson–White syndrome** (**Fig.** 12.7).

ECG characteristics

The electrocardiographic characteristics are within the P–QRS–T complex. There is a very short PR interval, a slur or notch (delta wave) in the upstroke of the R wave and a slight prolongation of the QRS complex, which can take on a wide and bizarre appearance (Fig. 12.8).

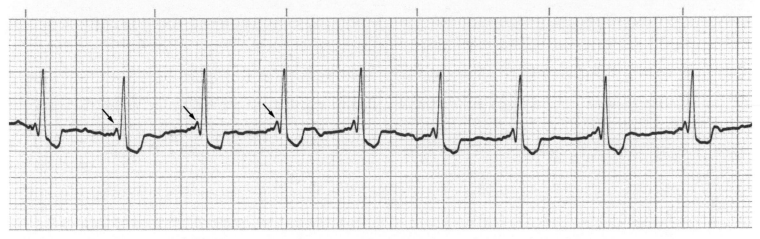

Figure 12.8 ECG from a Golden Retriever showing a very short P–R interval indicative of pre-excitation. P waves are arrowed; note how short the PR interval is. This indicates the presence of an accessory pathway and thus the potential for a rapid SVT (25 mm/s and 10 mm/mV).

PART 4
Management, clinical significance and treatment of arrhythmias

Chapter 13: Management of arrhythmias
Chapter 14: Clinical significance and treatment of tachyarrhythmias
Chapter 15: Clinical significance and treatment of bradyarrhythmias

13 • Management of arrhythmias

Arrhythmias are a frequent finding in cardiac diseases, but are also often secondary to systemic diseases. This chapter discusses the decision-making process as to when to treat arrhythmias.

Before using specific antiarrhythmic drugs, which have the potential to be pro-arrhythmic, two questions need to be answered (Fig. 13.1).

(1) Does the arrhythmia suggest the presence of an underlying condition?
(2) Is the arrhythmia of primary clinical significance?

1. Does the arrhythmia suggest the presence of an underlying condition?

This is important because the underlying condition may require treatment first, leading to a resolution (or reduction) in the arrhythmia. Possible underlying conditions can be broadly categorised into primary cardiac diseases and non-cardiac diseases.

Primary cardiac diseases

There is potential for any clinically significant cardiac disease to lead to myocardial stress, dilation or hypoxia, which can be a stimulus for arrhythmias. Typically, atrial dilation and stretch can lead to atrial arrhythmias such as supraventricular premature complexes and atrial fibrillation. Ventricular dilation or hypertrophy can lead to ventricular premature complexes. In general practice, mitral valve disease would be the most common cause of atrial dilation in dogs, leading to supraventricular arrhythmias, and cardiomyopathies would be a common cause of ventricular arrhythmias in both dogs and cats. In such cases it is important to initially manage and treat the heart failure, particularly if there are congestive failure signs prior to considering specific antiarrhythmic drugs.

A review of any concurrent antiarrhythmic drugs should also be considered as a possible iatrogenic cause of arrhythmias. For example, sotalol may lead to AV block, pimobendan may exacerbate arrhythmias associated with accessory pathways, digoxin may trigger ventricular arrhythmias, theophylline may result in supraventricular arrhythmias and sedative drugs can result in bradyarrhythmias.

However, there are some specific situations, that is, in Boxers and Dobermans, with dilated cardiomyopathy, in addition to the treatment for heart failure, antiarrhythmic drugs are considered appropriate to reduce the likelihood of sudden death (see later).

Non-cardiac diseases

There is a very long list of medical conditions that can trigger effects on the heart, leading to arrhythmias. These conditions may range from atrial standstill caused by hyperkalaemia to ventricular arrhythmias associated with splenic disease or gastric dilation (see AIVR in page 37) and from arrhythmias caused by hypoxia (e.g. due to respiratory disease) to

Small Animal ECGs: An Introductory Guide, Third Edition. Mike Martin.
© 2015 John Wiley & Sons, Ltd. Published 2015 by John Wiley & Sons, Ltd.

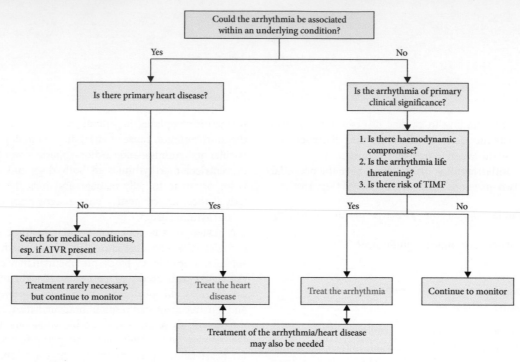

Figure 13.1 Flow chart summarising the decision-making process in treating an arrhythmia.

bradyarrhythmia associated with intracranial disease. When presented with an animal in which the diagnostic tests have not revealed the presence of a primary cardiac condition, then the search needs to be widened to include non-cardiac conditions, with a very thorough and comprehensive physical examination (and history) together with extensive blood profiles, urine analysis and radiography and/or ultrasonography to screen for non-cardiac diseases. In the vast majority of situations in which a non-cardiac disease has been found in association with an arrhythmia, treatment directed towards the condition will often lead to

a resolution of the arrhythmia. Simple monitoring of the arrhythmia may be all that is required in many cases, unless the arrhythmia is of primary significance. Additionally, monitoring of the arrhythmia can often be a good means to assess the response to treatment of the medical condition, for example, resolution of atrial standstill in dogs with Addison's disease.

It may be that arrhythmias develop as a consequence of medical drug therapy, and a review of all concurrent medications should be performed.

2. Is the arrhythmia of primary clinical significance?

An arrhythmia may be of primary clinical significance if it results in:

- signs of haemodynamic compromise,
- has the potential to lead to sudden death,
- could lead to heart failure (e.g. tachycardia-induced myocardial failure).

Arrhythmias causing haemodynamic compromise

Haemodynamic compromise, and thus clinical signs, will occur when an arrhythmia results in a significant reduction in cardiac output and often blood pressure. This can occur secondary to either profound bradyarrhythmias or sustained and rapid tachyarrhythmias.

Bradyarrhythmias

When the heart rate slows down, there is a natural compensatory increase in stroke volume to sustain cardiac output (Starling's Law of the heart), with the aim of sustaining blood pressure. However, if a bradycardia was profound, it would reach a point at which there would be an inability to compensate for the reduction in heart rate. Typically, dogs that have complete AV block with a heart rate of 30–40/min remain conscious and are able to walk into the clinic; however, heart rates lower than 25/min tend to start producing weakness or recumbency. Dogs with a sinus arrest pause of 20 seconds at rest may not necessarily faint; however, the same pause at exercise would result in syncope, reflecting the higher metabolic demand.

Tachyarrhythmias

With tachyarrhythmias, as the heart rate increases, there is less diastolic filling time, which consequently reduces the stroke volume and thus the cardiac output. The degree of reduction in stroke volume is greater with ventricular arrhythmias as compared with supraventricular arrhythmias. With a supraventricular arrhythmia, the depolarisation, and thus the contraction, of the left ventricle sustains a normal depolarisation sequence, therefore producing an efficient myocardial contraction. However, when there is a ventricular arrhythmia, depolarisation and contraction are inefficient and ejection of blood is not well coordinated, resulting in a reduction in stroke volume. Thus, a supraventricular tachycardia may not result in signs of forward failure and weakness or collapse until it exceeds 300/min, whereas a ventricular tachycardia may produce haemodynamic compromise at lower rates, sometimes as low as 200/min. The heart rate at which clinical signs of compromise occur will also be influenced by the presence of concurrent disease.

Note

It should be understood that occasional or even frequent arrhythmias are not likely to result in haemodynamic compromise. As a generalisation, there needs to be a sustained reduction in cardiac output to lower the blood pressure sufficiently to produce clinical signs, which will usually require a sustained arrhythmia.

Clinical signs of haemodynamic compromise

The clinical signs of haemodynamic compromise are essentially those of forward failure and low blood pressure, that is, reduced mental status, weak/poor pulse strength and mucosal pallor. In more severe cases, there may also be cold extremities. Blood pressure assessment (Fig. 13.2) is useful to check for hypotension, although it can often be difficult to obtain a blood pressure recording accurately in very hypotensive animals. Animals may also present with a history of syncope or pre-syncope, recumbency or even sudden death. In animals with a concurrent disease, whether cardiac or non-cardiac, it can sometimes be difficult to ascertain if the signs are necessarily due to the arrhythmia or the disease. This requires clinical judgement and experience.

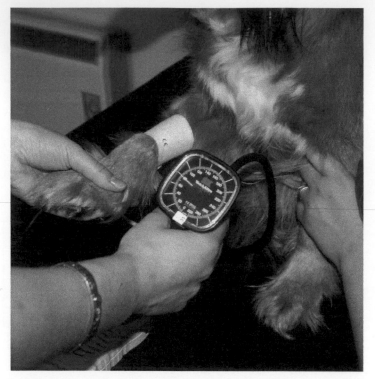

Figure 13.2 Photograph of an older dog having her blood pressure assessed. Measurement of blood pressure is particularly useful in dogs and cats with an arrhythmia to determine if the arrhythmia is causing hypotension or not. It is essential in any animal that presents in a state of weakness or collapse.

Note

Measurement of blood pressure is very useful in determining the haemodynamic significance of arrhythmias and should be considered a routine procedure in both the assessment and monitoring.

Life-threatening arrhythmias

As a general rule, a sustained and rapid ventricular tachycardia with hypotension is considered high risk of progression into ventricular fibrillation and results in death; thus rapid i/v cardioversion is normally performed. Additionally, very frequent and multimorphic ventricular arrhythmias are usually considered malignant and require drug suppression. Profound bradyarrhythmias, such as sinus arrest (or sick sinus syndrome) or AV block with an inconsistent and slow ventricular escape rhythm, are considered life-threatening and may require pacemaker implantation.

Tachycardia-induced myocardial failure (TIMF)

This occurs as a consequence of an incessant tachycardia sustained over a period of days or weeks. In dogs, this is most commonly seen with rapid sustained supraventricular tachycardias (Chapters 6 and 12). Myocardial failure develops, leading to signs of congestive heart failure, which can mimic dilated cardiomyopathy on echocardiographic examination. While it may not seem urgent in the first few days, if cardioversion is not successful, the relentless progression into heart failure makes this a challenging case to manage; thus, prompt cardioversion is preferable (by medication or ablation). Additionally, it can be useful to withdraw any positive dromotropic drugs, such as pimobendan, when managing these arrhythmias. The myocardial failure can be sustained for days or weeks following cardioversion to sinus rhythm.

Atrial fibrillation

Atrial fibrillation is most commonly associated with dilation and stretch of one or both atria, resulting in the inability to sustain the normal depolarisation sequence. In such cases, animals usually present with heart failure, and the sympathetic drive results in a rapid ventricular response rate with >50% pulse deficit. Control of the ventricular response rate (i.e. heart rate) is then desirable, minimising the pulse deficit. In dogs with myocardial disease, digoxin is considered the drug of choice (sometimes in combination with diltiazem); however, other options include calcium channel antagonists and β-blockers. In contrast, in giant-breed dogs that present with lone AF, that are, not in heart failure, it is debatable whether any treatment is required or not.

Note

When to treat arrhythmias is not an easy decision, but it is mostly based on experience with a good understanding of cardiology. Otherwise, it is prudent to seek advice from a Specialist in Cardiology or consider referral to them.

The decision on treatment of arrhythmias

Having made the decision that an arrhythmia is of primary significance, then antiarrhythmic drugs need to be chosen. However, it is still important to remember that antiarrhythmic drugs may have proarrhythmic effects and can complicate the arrhythmia; thus, continual monitoring and re-assessment are necessary. The aims of treatment also need to be considered in advance. It is often unlikely that animals with frequent ventricular arrhythmias will have a complete resolution of the arrhythmias following medication. Thus, judgement of the response should not be based on the ECG findings alone, but importantly on the clinical improvement in the animal with a reduction or resolution of the signs.

14 • Clinical significance and treatment of tachyarrhythmias

This chapter discusses the clinical significance and treatment of the more common tachyarrhythmias. Please note that the clinical findings (on examination and auscultation) are discussed in Chapters 5 and 6, together with the electrocardiographic features.

Sinus tachycardia

Clinical significance

Sinus tachycardia (Chapter 3) is a very common rhythm associated with excitement, exercise and stress. Thus, it is of paramount importance to evaluate the 'state' of the patient – during which an ECG recording may, of course, also cause a degree of stress and fear. Sinus tachycardia can also be seen with many medical conditions, for example, conditions associated with pyrexia, pain, anaemia, shock, dehydration, haemorrhage, septicaemia, toxaemia or hyperthyroidism. In addition, concurrent medications, sedatives or anaesthetics should also be taken into consideration. Hence sinus tachycardia is often a non-specific rhythm disturbance. However, it is also associated with heart failure, as a result of the compensatory sympathetic drive; whereas, dogs that do not have heart failure retain a normal respiratory sinus arrhythmia.

Treatment

Oftentimes, sinus tachycardia is not a primary rhythm disturbance, but secondary to another cause, whether it is physiological or medical;

therefore, antiarrhythmic drug treatment is usually not indicated. Treatment should be directed towards the primary cause, whether it is a medical condition or secondary to heart failure.

> **Note**
>
> In animals in congestive heart failure, a sinus tachycardia is often a necessary compensatory response in an attempt to maintain the cardiac output. Thus antiarrhythmic drugs are not used to slow down the heart rate – instead, treatment is directed towards the congestive heart failure, following which the heart rate usually slows down as the sympathetic drive reduces.

Supraventricular arrhythmias

Supraventricular premature complexes (SVPCs) and Supraventricular tachycardia (SVT)

Clinical significance

Supraventricular arrhythmias (Chapter 6) may be an indicator of underlying atrial disease, which would indicate the need for further diagnostic investigations such as echocardiography and thoracic radiography. The significance of supraventricular arrhythmias will depend on their frequency and the rate of a sustained SVT. Infrequent SVPCs do not

Small Animal ECGs: An Introductory Guide, Third Edition. Mike Martin.
© 2015 John Wiley & Sons, Ltd. Published 2015 by John Wiley & Sons, Ltd.

generally compromise the cardiac output and, therefore, often do not require treatment, but may be an indicator of underlying conditions; for example, they may be associated with:

- Primary heart disease that results in atrial dilation or stretch secondary to AV valve regurgitation, which may be associated with congenital or acquired AV valve defects (dysplasia or endocardiosis), cardiomyopathy or congenital cardiac shunts. Occasionally, it may be seen with heart base tumours such as a right atrial haemangiosarcoma.
- Some drugs such as: digitalis toxicity, 'stimulant-type' drugs such as theophylline or drugs with positive dromotropic properties such as pimobendan.
- Systemic illness, such as hyperthyroidism in cats.
- An elevation in sympathetic tone, which can be associated with stress or pain, for example.

Occasional SPVCs will not cause hypotension; however, a rapid SVT can result in haemodynamic compromise with hypotension (Table 14.2), and animals may present with exercise intolerance, lethargy, episodic weakness or recumbency. Clinical signs can be more severe when there is concurrent structural heart disease. When an SVT is maintained at a high rate (>250/min) for days or weeks, it can result in tachycardia-induced myocardial failure (TIMF) and congestive heart failure (which can mimic dilated cardiomyopathy).

Treatment

The aims of treatment are to improve the clinical signs and reduce the frequency or severity of episodic weakness associated with a sustained SVT. Infrequent SPVCs do not generally compromise the cardiac output or cause hypotension and, therefore, often do not require treatment; rather the treatment should be directed towards the underlying primary cause, which may additionally reduce the frequency of the SPVCs. In contrast, animals with a rapid SVT, resulting in hypotensive weakness, would require treatment. In addition, an elevated sympathetic

tone can exacerbate arrhythmias, whether it is related to stress or pain, for example, and management of this might be considered if present.

If SPVCs are considered frequent enough to be clinically significant, then oral medications (see the following text box) are likely to be the first line of choice such as: digoxin (if there is concurrent myocardial failure), diltiazem or β-blockers (such as atenolol or sotalol).

Oral supraventricular antiarrhythmic drugs

- Calcium antagonists
  - Diltiazem
    - dog: 0.5–3 mg/kg q8 hr
    - cat: 0.05–3 mg/kg q8 hr
  - Verapamil
    - dog: 0.5–3 mg/kg q8 hr
    - cat: 0.5–1 mg/kg q8 hr
- β-blockers
  - Atenolol
    - dog: 0.25–2 mg/kg q12 hr
    - cat: 6.25–12.5 mg per cat q12 hr
  - Propranolol
    - dog: 0.2–2 mg/kg q8 hr
    - cat: 2.5–5 mg per cat q8 hr
- Digoxin (drug of choice if there is ventricular myocardial failure)
  - Dose: see under Atrial fibrillation (AF)
- Sotalol
  - Dose
    - dog: 0.5–3 mg/kg q12 hr
    - cat: 10–20 mg per cat q12 hr
- Amiodarone (dog)
  - Dose – see separate text box under Ventricular Arrhythmias

---

When an SVT results in symptoms such as a dog presenting with recumbency or episodic weakness, then treatment is indicated. As discussed in Chapter 12, there are few recognised 'types' of SVT, namely focal atrial tachycardia (FAT), atrial flutter and orthodromic atrioventricular reciprocating tachycardia (OAVRT). The treatment of these differs, so a definitive diagnosis is important. If the SVT alternates between sinus rhythm and SVT, then diagnosis of the underlying rhythm might be ascertained (Chapter 12); however, if the SVT is sustained with no break in the rhythm, then the diagnosis is more difficult. One method is to try to interrupt the SVT, be it very briefly, by various techniques, such as a precordial thump, i/v drugs (such as lidocaine) and/or vagal manoeuvres.

A precordial thump to the left apex may induce a short break in the SVT, which can help determine the underlying rhythm. Rarely, this might induce a sustained cardioversion to a normal sinus rhythm.

The next step is to consider i/v drugs to either cardiovert the SVT to normal, or to induce a brief break of the SVT or slow down the SVT, which can provide an opportunity to examine the underlying rhythm. Often, the first drug of choice is lidocaine (see text box on lidocaine), which seems to work well on accessory pathways and thus often converts an OAVRT (a common cause of SVT in dogs). If lidocaine fails, then esmolol or verapamil would be the next drug to consider. Additionally, performing vagal manoeuvres after each drug is worth trying.

Vagal manoeuvres are techniques to attempt to profoundly increase the vagal tone and produce a marked slowing of the heart rate. This includes cold immersion to induce the diving reflex, for example. However, a common vagal manoeuvre used in dogs is carotid sinus massage. This is best performed when the dog is calm and there is no elevation in sympathetic tone. The carotid arteries are palpated bilaterally behind the angle of the jaw and then firm massaging pressure is applied for 5–10 seconds along the carotids. If effective, this will result in slowing of both the sinus and AV nodes, to potentially interrupt or slow down an SVT.

If there is cardioversion of an SVT to a normal rhythm, then whichever drug proved effective would be continued orally. However, there are often problems with long-term control of SVTs with oral antiarrhythmic drugs, most commonly the development of drug resistance (requiring increasing dosages), owner compliance issues or episodes of vomiting or diarrhoea resulting in lower blood levels of the drug. Radiofrequency ablation is now an option with good outcomes in dogs with an accessory pathway. This requires referral to a centre of excellence performing this procedure: undertaking electrophysiological studies to map where the accessory pathway is and then ablation of the pathway.

Response to the treatment can be assessed from Holter monitoring pre- and post-treatment. A significant response to antiarrhythmic drugs would be a significant reduction in sustained SVT, as well as the absence of clinical signs such as episodic weakness.

Intravenous supraventricular antiarrhythmic drugs

- Lidocaine – see text box under Ventricular Arrhythmias
- Esmolol – a short-acting β-blocker with a half-life of 9 min
  - Dose
    - dog: 0.05–0.5 mg/kg i/v over 5 min
    - cat: 0.05–0.5 mg/kg i/v over 5 min
- Verapamil
  - Dose
    - dog: 0.05 mg/kg i/v every 5 min to effect (max. 0.15 mg/kg in 10–15 min)

Radiofrequency ablation for OAVRT

This is now available in a few veterinary centres of excellence around the world, for the treatment of SVTs due to accessory pathways such as OAVRT. Most accessory pathways in dogs seem to be right-sided, which makes them more accessible for venous cardiac catheterisation. The accessory pathway is mapped using electrophysiological techniques, and then the pathway is ablated. This results in a 'cure' of the SVT when successful and initial outcomes are proving good. Referral of dogs with symptomatic SVTs should therefore be offered as an option to owners.

Atrial fibrillation

Clinical significance

AF (see also Chapter 6) is usually an indicator of underlying atrial disease, most commonly atrial dilation, which would indicate the need for further diagnostic investigations such as echocardiography and thoracic radiography. AF does not have major haemodynamic effects. The loss of the atrial contraction contribution to cardiac output is approximately 10–20%, which is compensated for primarily by an increase in rate and stroke volume. Since AF is most commonly seen in animals with atrial dilation, these animals often present with heart failure and thus have an elevated sympathetic drive, which produces a rapid ventricular response (i.e. high heart rate). AF can be associated with conditions such as:

- Dilation and stretching of one or both atria from a number of potential causes:
  - Dilated cardiomyopathy, typically in larger-breed dogs.
  - Mitral valve disease in any breed of dog, when the left atrium is markedly dilated.
  - It is uncommon in cats, but is sometimes seen when there is severe left atrial dilation with hypertrophic or restrictive cardiomyopathy.
  - AV valve regurgitation for any other cause that leads to marked atrial dilation such as mitral dysplasia or tricuspid dysplasia.
  - Other defects that result in atrial dilation such as patent ductus arteriosus, ventricular septal defect.
- Sometimes, it is seen in dogs with cardiac tumours.
- Occasionally, it is seen following rapid drainage of a pericardial effusion.

AF is occasionally also seen without evidence of atrial dilation; this is termed 'lone' AF, or sometimes referred to as **idiopathic AF**. This is more commonly seen in giant-breed dogs such as Irish Wolfhounds, Newfoundlands, Great Dane, Dogue de Bordeaux and Bull Mastiffs, but also in German Shepherd dogs. Lone AF usually has a fairly normal ventricular response rate (heart rate <120/min), as there is no increase in sympathetic drive because the dogs are not in heart failure. However, many giant-breed dogs with lone AF progress to dilated cardiomyopathy and ultimately heart failure. At present, there is no evidence for any benefit of treatment for dogs with lone AF.

Treatment

It must be remembered that AF is most commonly seen in animals that are also in congestive heart failure; so the treatment priority should be towards this.

Cardioversion of AF to sinus rhythm is generally not attempted because there is usually cardiac pathology, the success rate is low, and of the few that do convert, many relapse back into AF. If the AF is of very recent onset, for example, occurring following pericardiocentesis, then attempting cardioversion with i/v lidocaine is worth trying, although many of these cases will naturally revert back to sinus rhythm without treatment.

In dogs with underlying heart failure, which is the most common presentation in practice, the aim of treatment is to control the ventricular response rate by slowing down the AV nodal conduction. The convention is to achieve an in-clinic heart rate of less than 150/min. For most, the drug of choice for rate control of AF is digoxin, because of its mild positive inotropic properties. If there is good myocardial function, then calcium antagonists or β-blockers are alternative options; however, these should be used with caution in dogs with myocardial failure. If rate control is not satisfactory with digoxin alone, then combining it with diltiazem is considered the next option.

However, rate control is very difficult to measure in clinical practice. Holter monitoring of dogs has shown a marked elevation of the heart rate in dogs with or without AF while 'in the vets', as compared to the heart rate at home. Therefore, simply auscultating the heart rate in the clinic is not a reliable method of assessing heart rate control. Ideally, Holter monitors need to be used to achieve this, although this can become cost prohibitive for some owners. It is still not clear how important aggressive heart rate control is in AF and whether rate control produces better clinical outcomes. A more pragmatic approach is to place more emphasis on the clinical status of the dog, as opposed to solely on the heart rate.

Use of digoxin for rate control of AF

Digoxin dose

Primarily used in dogs; indications for use in cats are rare.

- Dose in dog = $0.22 \, \text{mg/m}^2$ every 12 hours; however, Table 14.1 provides a simplified guideline for a starting dose
- Dose in cat: <4 kg – 0.0625 mg tablet 1/2 q48h and >4 kg – 0.0625 mg tablet 1/2 q24h (however, this is rarely ever used in cats)

Steady-state levels are achieved in 5–7 days. Serum digoxin levels should be measured (approximately 6–8 hours post pill) to confirm the dose is correct, as it varies between individual patients. Therapeutic dose range is 0.8–2.5 ng/ml; 1–2 ng/ml is a good target.

Causes of a persistent high heart rate in dogs with AF.

- Elevation of the heart rate in-clinic due to nervousness at the time of examination; this would require 24 hour Holter to determine the average heart rate at home.
- Inadequate control of the congestive failure signs; such that the sympathetic drive is still high.
- Dehydration or hypotension due to over-diuresis or vasodilation.
- Inadequate serum therapeutic levels of digoxin.
- Concurrent medical disease, for example, renal failure.
- Advanced myocardial failure and end-stage heart disease.
- Heart rate poorly responsive to digoxin (check with 24 hour Holter) – may require additional antiarrhythmic drug such as diltiazem.

Table 14.1   Digoxin starting dose in dogs.

Body weight	Tablet size	Tablet dose
1–5 kg	62.5 µg (PG)	1/2 q12 hr
6–13 kg	62.5 µg (PG)	1 q12 hr
14–23 kg	125 µg	1 q12 hr
24–36 kg	125 µg	1 1/2 q12 hr
>37 kg	250 µg	1 q12 hr

Note: The dose in Dobermans is 125 µg tablet 1 q12 h.

Bioaccumulation may occur with: azotaemia, low serum albumin, or cachexia. Signs of overdosage (digoxin toxicity) typically develop after 2–4 days following commencement of digoxin (or after an increase in dose). The most common signs are: depression, anorexia, vomiting, diarrhoea and arrhythmias; in which case, the drug should be stopped and re-introduced (after a couple of days) at a lower dose when the signs have resolved.

Ventricular arrhythmias

Ventricular premature complexes (VPCs) and Ventricular tachycardia (VT)

Clinical significance

Ventricular arrhythmias (Chapter 5) may be an indicator of underlying disease (cardiac or non-cardiac) and that disease may be of greater clinical importance than the arrhythmia. The significance of ventricular arrhythmias will depend on their frequency and complexity. There is potentially a marked range in frequency and severity of ventricular arrhythmias from a few VPCs to a sustained VT. Infrequent VPCs may

Table 14.2 Guidelines on the assessment of systemic hypotension from systolic blood pressure measurement.

Normal	>120 mmHg
Borderline hypotension	100–120 mmHg
Hypotension	<100 mmHg
Severe hypotension	<90 mmHg
Life-threatening hypotension	<80 mmHg

not result in haemodynamic compromise but may be an indicator of underlying disease; for example, they may be associated with:

- Primary heart disease such as: cardiomyopathy (particularly in Dobermans and Boxers), inherited ventricular arrhythmia syndrome in young GSDs, myocarditis (e.g. traumatic myocarditis/contusion), cardiac neoplasia, endocarditis, myocardial infarction or ischaemia in cats secondary to thromboembolic disease.
- Low blood oxygen saturation, for example, hypoxia associated with congestive heart failure or respiratory diseases.
- Drugs such as digitalis, anaesthetics, atropine and isoprenaline.
- A systemic disorder (see also accelerated idioventricular rhythm page 113) such as: gastric dilation, pancreatitis, splenic masses, electrolyte imbalance, uraemia, pyometra and snake bites (e.g. adders).

Occasional VPCs will not cause hypotension, whereas a rapid and sustained VT can result in haemodynamic compromise with hypotension (Table 14.2) and thus signs such as: pallor, exercise intolerance, weakness/recumbency or syncope. When the ventricular arrhythmia is a very fast VT with R-on-T, the risk of developing ventricular fibrillation (VF) and sudden death is considered high and would warrant antiarrhythmic drug treatment. If a dog has a history of syncope with the documentation of a high number of VPCs, with complexity, on Holter, then institution of antiarrhythmic drugs may be considered. However, be aware that some dogs may present with both bradyarrhythmia, such as intermittent sinus arrest, and VPCs, and it can be difficult to decide which was the cause of the syncope.

> **Note**
>
> In animals with a history of collapse, a definitive diagnosis can only be made if the animal collapses while wearing a Holter, to document whether it was a tachyarrhythmia or bradyarrhythmia that was the cause of the collapse.

The frequency and complexity of ventricular arrhythmias are best assessed by Holter monitoring. In assessing the severity of ventricular arrhythmias from a 24 hour Holter monitor, both the frequency and the complexity of the VPCs are important (Table 14.3). VT, frequent multiform (polymorphic) VPCs and increasing complexity, such as pairs, triplets, runs and R-on-T, are usually considered to represent severe and potentially life-threatening arrhythmias that might warrant antiarrhythmic drug treatment. Very fast VT, with R-on-T, has the highest risk of development of VF and sudden death. In Dobermans, a sustained ventricular tachycardia (VT) >30 seconds is considered a predictor of sudden death.

Treatment

The aims of treatment are to improve clinical signs, reduce the risk of sudden death and reduce the frequency and severity of syncope. However, when to commence antiarrhythmic drug treatment is ill-defined, and while this may be dictated by the clinical presentation, it is often based on the experience and opinion of the cardiologist. Infrequent VPCs do not generally compromise the cardiac output or cause hypotensive events and, therefore, usually do not require treatment;

Table 14.3 A guideline on the classification[1] of ventricular arrhythmias on Holter monitoring, when considering antiarrhythmic therapy. This can be based on a combination of the number of VPCs per 24 h and the complexity of the ventricular arrhythmia.

Severity	Number of VPCs per 24 h	Complexity
Normal	<50	Single VPCs, monomorphic
Mild	50–1000	Pairs and triplets, non-sustained runs of VT, mostly monomorphic.
Moderate	1000–10000	The above + sustained runs of VT, often polymorphic.
Severe	>10000	The above + Sustained runs of very fast VT often with R-on-T, polymorphic VPCs or VT

[1]There are no specific publications or agreement to define severity; this is a simplified guideline based on the author's experience, with the aims of providing some guidance to the practitioner.

rather, treatment should be directed towards the underlying primary cause. In contrast, animals with a rapid VT, in which there is a marked reduction in cardiac output and hypotension, would warrant treatment. The first steps are to decide how severe the ventricular arrhythmia is (see Holter severity classification table 14.3) and if it is associated with concurrent cardiac, or non-cardiac, disease that might warrant treatment initially. Treatment of the primary underlying cause (e.g. congestive heart failure) will often produce a significant reduction in VPCs; thus, in many cases, antiarrhythmic drugs might be postponed to see if this occurs. In addition, an elevated sympathetic tone can exacerbate arrhythmias, whether it is related to stress or pain, for example, and management of this might be considered if present.

> ## Indications for antiarrhythmic drug treatment of ventricular arrhythmias
>
> - Classified as severe, on 24 hour Holter monitoring, in any breed
> - Classified as moderate or severe, on 24 hour Holter monitoring, in Boxers, Dobermans or young GSDs with inherited ventricular arrhythmia syndrome, or any breed with concurrent cardiomyopathy or myocarditis.

Additionally, some studies have shown that antiarrhythmic drugs have the potential to cause sudden death (i.e. proarrhythmic); thus their use needs strong justification. In most circumstances, institution of antiarrhythmics orally is satisfactory.

If VPCs are life-threatening, i/v lidocaine is often the drug of choice (see the following boxed text).

Following cardioversion of a ventricular arrhythmia with lidocaine, the options are as follows:

- Wait and see if the arrhythmia does return – in which case, repeat cardioversion is required.
- Medicate with an oral antiarrhythmic, which seems the most pragmatic approach.
- Administer i/v lidocaine as a constant rate infusion,
  - Usual starting dose is 50 µg/kg/min.
  - Steady-state levels take 3–6 hr to reach, and thus, small boluses of lidocaine may be required in the interim.
- If i/v lidocaine proves ineffective, then an alternative i/v option is esmolol.

Lidocaine (lignocaine)

- Drug of choice for the cardioversion of acute life-threatening VT.
- Its effects are nullified in the presence of hypokalaemia.
- Following i/v administration, the half-life is approximately 60–90 min in dogs (a lot longer in cats), but antiarrhythmic effects wane after 10 min.

Dosage

- Dog: i/v dose at 2–3 mg/kg boluses, every 3 min, max. of 9 mg/kg in 20 min.
- Cat: Slow i/v at 0.25–0.75 mg/kg, may give a repeat i/v injection after 20 min.

Toxicity

Note: cats are prone to toxicity (seizures and respiratory arrest).

- Signs of toxicity are neurological (twitching, nystagmus, seizures); these are usually self-limiting and gastrointestinal (nausea, vomiting, salivation).
- Airway obstruction and/or respiratory arrest in cats following seizures.
- Control seizures with i/v diazepam – 0.1 mg/kg i/v, repeat every few minutes to effect (max. 0.3 mg/kg) + elevate head.

If the ventricular arrhythmia is not imminently life-threatening, then antiarrhythmics can be commenced orally. Mexiletine has been one of the most common antiarrhythmics used in dogs; however, it is no longer manufactured. Thus, many have switched to using sotalol as the first drug of choice; but it seems to have less overall success compared to mexiletine. Sotalol has also been used more often as the first antiarrhythmic drug of choice for the treatment of Boxer cardiomyopathy. However, there are other drug options – see the following text box. Amiodarone is a newer drug finding increasing use, but is usually only considered if other options have been unsatisfactory,

as it is a difficult drug to use and requires considerable monitoring. β-blockers are the drugs most commonly used to control ventricular arrhythmias in cats.

Oral ventricular antiarrhythmic drugs

- Sotalol
  - dog: 0.5–2.0 mg/kg q12 hr
- Atenolol
  - dog: 0.5–2 mg/kg q12 hr
  - cat: 2 mg/kg q12–24 hr
- Mexiletine
  - dog: 5–8 mg/kg q8 hr *per os*
- Propranolol
  - dog: 0.2–2.0 mg/kg q8 hr
  - cat: 2.5 mg q8–12 hr
- Magnesium amino chelate (200 mg tablets) at 10 mg/kg daily with food
- Amiodarone (dogs) – see below

Amiodarone (dogs)

- Reported to have significant side effects, so tends to be used as a last resort.
- Need to monitor liver and thyroid function regularly.
- Loading dose: 10 mg/kg q12 hr for 1 week.
- Maintenance dose: 5–7.5 mg/kg q24 hr.
- Serum levels should be measured weekly until steady-state levels are achieved, thereafter every 2–4 months.

Response to treatment can be assessed from Holter monitoring pre- and post-treatment. A significant response to antiarrhythmic drugs is considered to be a reduction in VPCs by 75% when the VPCs are frequent. But probably more important is the suppression of fast VT, particularly if associated with R-on-T.

Ventricular arrhythmias associated with GDV

Approximately 40%–50% of dogs with gastric dilatation volvulus (GDV) develop ventricular arrhythmias (often AIVR), 12–72 hr after the onset of GDV.

It is caused by:

- Myocardial ischaemia (decreased coronary perfusion)
- Reperfusion injury
- Hypokalaemia (can also make the arrhythmias resistant to antiarrhythmic drugs)
- Acidosis
- Hypoxia
- Myocardial depressant factors

Treatment is, therefore, directed towards:

- The shock and maintenance of normal hydration status;
- Correction of acid–base and electrolyte imbalances;
- Monitoring Na and K regularly in such cases is very useful as hypokalaemia is a common problem (although measurement of serum K may not reflect total body K).

Accelerated idioventricular rhythm (AIVR)

Clinical significance

AIVR (Chapter 5), sometimes given the nickname a 'slow VT', is usually not associated with primary heart disease, but non-cardiac medical conditions. AIVR is generally a transient rhythm (although it may persist for some days) rarely causing haemodynamic instability or requiring treatment and is usually well tolerated due to its slow ventricular rate. It is self-limiting and resolves as the sinus rate surpasses the rate of AIVR. It would be rare that AIVR would degenerate into VT or VF. However, misdiagnosis of AIVR as VT or complete heart block can lead to inappropriate therapies with potential complications. AIVR is often a clue to certain underlying conditions – in particular, various abdominal or medical conditions in dogs, such as gastric dilation, pancreatitis, splenic masses, electrolyte imbalance, reperfusion and hypoxia.

Treatment

The most important therapy for patients with AIVR is to treat the underlying aetiology.

- AIVR is usually haemodynamically well tolerated and self-limiting; thus, it rarely requires antiarrhythmic treatment.
- Continued ECG and blood pressure monitoring is important as it is possible for a dog to develop complications with true VT.
- In rare situations, atropine can be used to increase the underlying sinus rate to inhibit AIVR; however, there is some debate over the value of this approach.

Ventricular fibrillation (VF)

Clinical significance

VF results in absence of any effective ventricular contractions with a rapid fall in blood pressure, usually leading to death. The causes are numerous, but not dissimilar to those of VPCs and VT.

Treatment

Direct current electrical defibrillation is required to stop VF. This should only be performed when an animal is unconscious – which is likely to occur rapidly after the onset of VF. This needs to be performed as quickly as possible, even before other aspects of cardiopulmonary resuscitation (CPR) are started, as any delay in electrical defibrillation is associated with a reduced chance of success. However, the outcome will also depend on the extent of the existing pathology. The starting energy setting for external electrical defibrillation is approximately 4 Joules/kg. Three to four shocks are then administrated in quick succession and with increasing energy settings (usually increasing the machine setting by one notch after each attempt) until VF is stopped. It is hoped there is then a return of a sinus rhythm or another rhythm that produces ventricular contractions and improvement in blood pressure. CPR should then be continued as required.

15 • Clinical significance and treatment of bradyarrhythmias

This chapter discusses the clinical significance and treatment of the more common bradyarrhythmias. Please note that the clinical findings (on examination and auscultation) are discussed in Chapter 7, together with the electrocardiographic features.

Sinus bradycardia

Clinical significance

Sinus bradycardia (Chapter 3) is a very common rhythm associated with sleep or rest. It is of paramount importance to consider the 'state' of the patient; this would primarily affect the recordings obtained from a Holter monitor. Sinus bradycardia can also be seen in athletically fit breeds, particularly working dogs such as Border collies, Springer spaniels and Labradors. Sinus bradycardia can be associated with: hypothyroidism, hyperkalaemia, hypothermia, elevated intracranial pressure (e.g. following cranial trauma), systemic disease (e.g. renal failure) or drugs (tranquillisers or antiarrhythmic drugs) and, additionally in cats, feline dysautonomia. Cats sometimes present with a sinus bradycardia when presenting with heart failure, which seems paradoxical, since one of the compensatory responses to heart failure is an increase in sympathetic tone (i.e. a sinus tachycardia would be expected).

Treatment

If the sinus bradycardia is considered normal for the individual, then no treatment is indicated. However, if it is abnormal, then treatment should be aimed at the primary cause and investigations need to be performed to screen for these differentials. Vagolytic or beta-agonist drugs can be used to increase the heart rate if symptomatic, but this is rarely necessary.

Sinus arrest

Clinical significance

Sinus arrest can be a normal finding on a Holter recording of animals during sleep and are often referred to as sinus pauses, rather than sinus arrest. It is often considered a normal-variant in brachycephalic dogs, particularly if they have a degree of airway obstruction (i.e. exaggerated respiratory sinus arrhythmia).

Small Animal ECGs: An Introductory Guide, Third Edition. Mike Martin.
© 2015 John Wiley & Sons, Ltd. Published 2015 by John Wiley & Sons, Ltd.

A long period of sinus arrest may result in **syncope,** as no blood flows to the brain, blood pressure falls and fainting occurs. How long the period of sinus arrest must be to result in syncope depends on the activity (or metabolic rate) of the animal at the time; for example, a 5 second pause may be sufficient when running, but it may require 15–25 seconds at rest. **Pre-syncope** occurs if the duration of the sinus arrest is not quite sufficient to result in collapse but does cause signs of weakness or ataxia.

There are several conditions that may be associated with sinus arrest that overlap with causes of sinus bradycardia:

- Vagal stimulation associated with severe respiratory disease or associated with a vasovagal response, for example, with vomiting or tenesmus.
- Atrial disease such as dilation, fibrosis, cardiomyopathy or neoplasia (e.g. haemangiosarcoma and heart base tumours).
- Metabolic or endocrine diseases such as an electrolyte imbalance or hypothyroidism.
- Drugs, either due to their effects or associated with toxicity, must also be considered.
- Irritation of the vagus nerve by neoplasia in the cervical area (e.g. thyroid carcinoma) or in the thorax (e.g. aortic body tumour). Surgical manipulation within the thorax may also result in sinus arrest.
- Profound and regular sinus arrest can be a feature of sick sinus syndrome.

Treatment

Investigations need to be performed to screen for all of these differentials and treatment directed towards any underlying cause. If the sinus arrest is idiopathic, treatment is usually only required in symptomatic cases, such as those with a history of episodic weakness, presyncope or syncope. There is no satisfactory drug treatment, although many do try vagolytic drugs or beta-agonists. Pacemaker implantation is the treatment of choice, which will pace the heart during periods of sinus arrest and thus maintain blood pressure and prevent syncope as well as reduce the risk of sudden death.

> ### Neurally mediated syncope
>
> The most common form seems to be vasovagal syncope in dogs. This is thought to be due to an abnormal response to sudden excitement, often from rest, resulting in a vagal over-response to baroreceptors within the ventricles. This results in a combination of an inappropriate reflex vasodilation (vasodepressor) and bradycardia (cardioinhibition). This often seems to occur more frequently, or at times, when there is concurrent gastrointestinal or abdominal disease, or when bitches are in season.
>
> Holter monitoring, in association with the aforementioned diary-history, often shows an initial sinus tachycardia (with the excitement) and then a sudden inappropriate bradyarrhythmia, which is typically a period of sinus arrest or profound sinus bradycardia. One management option is to avoid the excitement triggers, but also to screen for the underlying medical conditions. In dogs with persistent syncope with no underlying cause, pacemaker implantation can help by pacing the heart during the period of bradyarrhythmia to sustain a normal heart rate. However, it does not counter the vasodilatory component. In most cases, the severity of the syncope following pacemaker is markedly reduced.

Sick sinus syndrome (sinus node dysfunction)

Clinical significance

As for sinus arrest described earlier, prolonged periods of no cardiac output will result in fall in blood pressure and, therefore, pre-syncope or syncope. A profound sinus bradycardia may present with lethargy and exercise intolerance due to an inability to increase the cardiac output on demand. In the bradycardia–tachycardia syndrome, either the bradycardia or the tachycardia may produce a significant drop in blood pressure and result in weakness or syncope, although the profound sinus bradycardia or sinus arrest is the most common cause of collapse. It is most commonly seen in West Highland White Terriers (with or without idiopathic pulmonary fibrosis); it has also been reported in older, female miniature Schnauzers. It has not been recorded in cats.

Treatment

If atropine (see the following boxed text) or exercise fails to increase the heart rate significantly, it would suggest that excessive vagal tone is not the cause of the bradycardia; this is considered a feature of sick sinus syndrome. It is usually difficult to obtain satisfactory rate control with medical treatment alone, although many do try vagolytic drugs or beta-agonists. The treatment of choice for symptomatic cases is pacemaker implantation. Rarely the tachycardia would also require antiarrhythmic drugs after pacing.

Atropine response test

Inject 40 µg/kg s/c (in dogs and cats) and re-assess the heart rate response by ECG in 30–40 minutes. A good response is considered an increase in heart rate by 100% or a heart rate of 150/min. A positive response is considered to be indicative of high vagal tone; in contrast, sinus node disease has a poor response. However, this is not a reliable test in animals and therefore, in practical terms, is not particularly useful.

Atrial standstill

Clinical significance

Atrial standstill is associated with two conditions in animals: hyperkalaemia and atrial cardiomyopathy. Clinical signs include weakness, lethargy, syncope and congestive heart failure.

Atrial standstill secondary to hyperkalaemia is reversible in response to appropriate treatment and so is sometimes referred to as **temporary** atrial standstill. Hyperkalaemia can be associated with conditions such as: Addison's disease (hypoadrenocorticism), diabetic ketoacidosis, oliguric renal failure, blocked urethra or extensive muscle trauma; there will also be additional clinical signs with these conditions. Iatrogenic causes include excessive potassium infusion or transfusion of stored blood. Digitalis toxicity is a rare cause that can be established from the history and measurement of serum levels.

Atrial cardiomyopathy is secondary to atrial disease usually affecting both atria (but can sometimes affect only the left atrium), resulting in congestive heart failure signs. The clinical signs are usually weakness, lethargy and syncope associated with the reduction in cardiac output and inability to increase the heart rate during activity. Congestive heart failure usually ensues insidiously and progressively. This condition is irreversible and sometimes referred to as **persistent** atrial standstill. Atrial cardiomyopathy, with atrial standstill, seems more prevalent is certain breeds: Cavalier King Charles Spaniels, English Springer Spaniels, Old English Sheepdogs, Italian Spinone, Labradors and mixed-breed dogs.

Atrial standstill can occur in association with a 'dying' heart and is termed **terminal atrial standstill.**

Treatment

Atrial standstill secondary to hyperkalaemia needs appropriate medical investigations and treatment; there is usually no need for additional 'cardiac' medications in these cases.

Persistent atrial standstill secondary to atrial cardiomyopathy is poorly responsive to any antiarrhythmic medication, including atropine; however, treatment should be directed towards congestive failure if present. The response to pacemaker implantation is mixed, with some dogs appearing to respond well with an extended quality of life (usually requiring ongoing heart failure medications), but in many cases, the heart failure remains progressive.

AV (heart) block

The clinical signs depend upon the severity of the heart block and the rate of any escape rhythm. Advanced second-degree and complete heart block are usually associated with clinical signs, whereas first-degree and mild second-degree heart blocks are not.

First-degree AV block

Clinical significance

First-degree block does not, in itself, cause any clinical problems. It may occur normally in an animal with a slow heart rate or in ageing animals due to degenerative changes in the AV node. Other causes include digitalis toxicity or other drugs such as propranolol or sotalol. It may occur when there is an abnormal potassium level. Treatment should be aimed at correcting the underlying cause.

Second-degree AV block

Mobitz type II

Clinical significance

Advanced cases of second-degree AV block may present with weakness, lethargy or syncope; it depends on the severity of the heart block, the resultant overall slow heart rate and the consequent reduction in cardiac output. Auscultation reveals an intermittent pause in the cardiac rhythm. Second-degree AV block that is severe or advanced (meaning the block occurs frequently) is usually Mobitz type II. It is this type that often progresses to complete AV block. Second-degree AV block (Mobitz type I) is often associated with low-grade AV block (infrequently dropped P waves).

Mobitz type I, second-degree AV block is sometimes seen in normal dogs with sinus arrhythmia, often on Holter recordings during sleep. It is often also seen in brachycephalic breeds with airway obstruction causing an exaggerated respiratory sinus arrhythmia. In these, both dropped P waves and short sinus arrest pauses are often present and are of no clinical significance.

Mobitz type II, second-degree AV block has been reported in older dogs with AV nodal fibrosis and hereditary stenosis of the bundle of His in Pugs; however, most cases are idiopathic. It may also occur with digitalis toxicity or other drugs, such as sotalol, xylazine, detomidine, atropine and quinidine, or with a potassium imbalance. The author is also aware of some anecdotal reports of heart block in dogs with hypothyroidism and hypoadrenocorticism.

Treatment

See complete heart block in the following section.

Complete heart block

Clinical significance

The clinical signs may include weakness, lethargy, syncope or sudden death, depending on how slow the ventricular rate is, and the subsequent reduction in cardiac output. A very slow ventricular escape rhythm is usually associated with more marked clinical signs, with the possibility of sudden death. It is common in chronic cases, with a slow ventricular response rate, to find a generalised cardiomegaly with or without evidence of congestive heart failure on thoracic radiography. On auscultation, a characteristic finding is a very regular and steady but slow heart beat together with the palpation of a hyperdynamic femoral pulse. In some cases, the more rapid atrial contraction sounds may be faintly audible. Complete AV block can be associated with cardiomyopathy, cardiac neoplasia, digitalis toxicity, AV node fibrosis, endocarditis, electrolyte imbalance (such as hypoadrenocorticism), hypothyroidism and Lyme disease. In cats, additionally, heart block is often association with the underlying structural heart disease such as restrictive or hypertrophic cardiomyopathy.

Treatment

In the past, treatment has often been attempted with parasympatholytic drugs (atropine, propantheline), sympathomimetic drugs (clenbuterol, terbutaline) or theophylline. However, currently the author favours pimobendan, which is a positive dromotrope (increases the rate of conduction through the electrical conduction tissue of the heart). In addition, the positive inotropic properties assist with ventricular emptying of a bradycardic heart.

In cats, millophyline may be of some help, and it would be rare to consider pacemaker implantation as few cases are idiopathic and many have an underlying cardiomyopathy.

In dogs, because heart block is commonly idiopathic (with no underlying structural heart disease), then pacemaker implantation is indicated, which provides symptomatic relief and reduces the risk of sudden death.

Drug doses

Inodilator

- Pimobendan : dog/cat : 0.1–0.3 mg/kg bid

Parasympatholytic drugs

- Atropine: dog/cat: 20–60 µg/kg q6–8 h *per os*
- Propantheline: dog: 0.5–2 mg/kg q8–12 h; cat: 7.5 mg q8–12 h *per os*

Sympathomimetic drugs

- Clenbuterol: dog: 1–5 µg/kg q8–12 h; cat 1 µg/kg q12–24 h
- Terbutaline: 1.25–5 mg per dog q8 h; 1.25 mg per cat q8 h

Pacemakers

Indications for pacemaker implantation

Any bradyarrhythmia resulting in clinical signs such as:

- Syncope
- Vasovagal syncope
- Presyncope
- Episodic weakness
- Exercise intolerance

Bradyarrhythmias

- Complete heart block
- Advanced second-degree heart block
- Sinus arrest
- Sick sinus syndrome
- Persistent atrial standstill

Contraindications

- Active infection, particularly pyoderma at the operation site
- Underlying structural heart disease such as cardiomyopathy or neoplasia

---

Bundle branch block

Right bundle branch block

Clinical significance

The right bundle branch (RBB) is long and slender thus vulnerable to damage. RBBB is not uncommon in normal healthy dogs but can be associated with congenital or acquired heart disease, cardiac neoplasia and trauma. RBBB can also be seen in association with Ashman's phenomenon (Chapter 11). RBBB, in itself, does not cause any significant haemodynamic problems.

Left bundle branch block

Clinical significance

The left bundle branch is thick, and therefore a larger lesion is required to produce conduction block. LBBB is therefore rare in normal healthy animals, and when it does occur, it is often associated with pathology: congenital (e.g. subaortic stenosis) or acquired heart disease (e.g.

hypertrophic or dilated cardiomyopathy), myocardial ischaemia, cardiac neoplasia or trauma. In itself, it does not cause any significant haemodynamic problems.

Left anterior fascicular block

Clinical significance

LAFB is often considered a relatively specific indicator of left ventricular myocardial disease in cats but can be seen with many heart diseases. It can be associated with hypertrophic or restrictive cardiomyopathy and electrolyte imbalance such as hyperkalaemia.

PART 5
Recording and interpreting ECGs

It is important to develop, and use, a routine when reading ECGs. Always read an ECG from its beginning, that is, from left to right. When the ECG is difficult to read, start from the easiest part of the tracing that is recognisable, then continue reading (left to right) from that point.

It is important to not over-interpret or be too dependent on ECG findings. Since the ECG records only the electrical activity of the heart, it should be remembered that this limits the information that can be gained from it. It is often poorly related to the mechanical function of the heart and does not provide information about aetiology or severity of structural heart disease. A normal ECG does not necessarily infer that the heart is normal and, likewise, an abnormal ECG is not necessarily indicative of heart disease. Additionally, if the ECG is abnormal, it is important to determine what the clinical significance is, and if treatment is indicated or not (Chapters 13, 14 and 15).

There are essentially four steps in ECG interpretation: rate, rhythm, complex measurement and mean electrical axis (Chapter 10). Of these, rate and rhythm are the most important and clinically relevant.

Calculate the heart rate

The heart rate is given in beats per minute. For the clinician, this should be fairly easy, as you have already examined the animal and determined the heart rate on auscultation. (!)

The heart rate varies from beat to beat, so the heart rate per minute is an average over that time period. The most accurate way, therefore, to count the heart rate would be to count a full minute; however, this is considered impractical on an ECG tracing. So a simpler method is to mark a 6-second strip of a representative part of the tracing. Count the number of complexes and multiply by 10. If the P wave rate and QRS–T complex rates differ, then record these separately.

A method for the mathematician

If there is not a 6 second strip, or if there is a short paroxysmal tachycardia, then the heart rate can be calculated from the P–P or R–R interval as follows. At a paper speed of 25 mm/s, there is 1500 mm per minute. Measure the distance, with a ruler, between two complexes (or count the number of small 1 mm boxes).

Small Animal ECGs: An Introductory Guide, Third Edition. Mike Martin.
© 2015 John Wiley & Sons, Ltd. Published 2015 by John Wiley & Sons, Ltd.

Heart rate (in beats per minute):

$$\text{HR (at 25 mm/s)} = \frac{1500}{\text{R} - \text{R interval (mm)}}$$

At a paper speed of 50 mm/s, there is 3000 mm per minute, thus:

$$\text{HR (at 50 mm/s)} = \frac{3000}{\text{R} - \text{R interval (mm)}}$$

However, the beat-to-beat measurement, which is the technique employed with 'ECG rulers', is considered the least accurate method of assessing the heart rate *per minute* because of the variation. An instantaneous rate is often very different (and variable) to the rate over a full minute.

Determine the rhythm

Generally, the author's approach is to look for the 'normal' QRS complexes first, which are usually recognisable as being tall and narrow. Then look to see if these are followed by T waves and preceded by P waves on every occasion.

Identifying parts of the ECG complex

In some instances, it can be difficult to identify the P waves, or it can be difficult to determine which are the P waves and which are the T waves (especially at fast heart rates).

Tip

It is often useful to mark the position of each P wave and QRS–T complex. This can be done by placing a piece of paper below the ECG tracing and placing a mark for each P and QRS (Fig. 16.1). This can help establish if there is a pattern, or if there are hidden complexes, and if a complex has occurred before or after it was due (or expected to occur).

Since the heart must always repolarise (to be depolarised again), there must always be a T wave following every QRS complex.

Using callipers, note the P–R interval and Q–T interval; for a run of beats, this will often reveal which deflection must be which – as the P–R and Q–T intervals will generally remain fairly constant. This method is most usefully performed on a stretch of ECG in which there is a variation in rate.

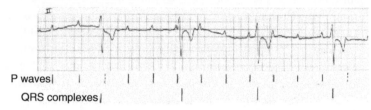

P waves|

QRS complexes|

Figure 16.1 ECG demonstrating how to mark out P waves and QRS complexes to help identify complexes. Note that the dotted lines represent hidden P waves – note how the first one changes the shape of the ST segment as compared with the others.

Measure the complex amplitudes and intervals

This is usually performed on a lead II rhythm strip at 50 mm/s on an unfiltered section. At 50 mm/s, 1 mm box = 0.02 s. Note the calibration.

Record the following (Fig. 16.2):

- P wave amplitude and duration
- R wave amplitude and QRS duration
- P–R interval – from start of P to start of QRS (strictly P–Q interval)
- Q–T interval – from start of QRS to end of T wave
- Note T wave morphology
- Note S–T segment elevation or depression

Use the table of normal values (Chapter 8) to check if the measurements are within normal values or not.

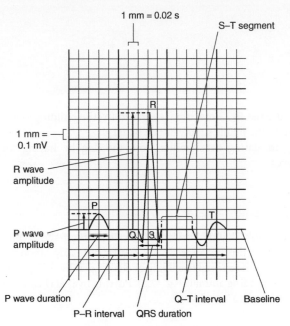

Figure 16.2 A schematic P–QRS–T complex (lead II) from a normal dog, illustrating the various amplitudes, durations and intervals (50 mm/s and 10 mm/mV).

17 • Artefacts

Artefacts are abnormal deflections reproduced on an ECG recording that are not associated with the electrical activity of the heart. They have the potential to either mask the ECG or mimic the ECG activity: producing an artefact-free tracing is therefore of paramount importance.

Electrical interference

Electrical interference produces fine, rapid and regular movements on the baseline of the ECG recording (Fig. 17.1). They can be associated with interference due to electrical cables (electromagnetic waves) within the room in which the recording is being made. They can be transmitted by the person restraining the animal who acts as an aerial or through the power-line of the ECG machine. The fine deflections usually occur at a rate of 50 per second (Hz) (60 per second in America). In the vast majority of instances, this artefact is associated with inadequate clip-to-skin contact.

To correct this problem:

- Ensure the clip-to-skin connections are good and are insulated (isolated); poor connections will permit electrical interference to manifest.
- Ensure the animal is insulated from the surface by placing a rug under it.

- Ensure the ECG machine is earthed (to the building), or try not to run on the mains supply but on battery.
- Try insulating the handler from the dog by having them wear gloves.

Muscle tremor artefact

This can look slightly similar to electrical interference, but the fine deflections in this instance are not regular but fairly random. It can be produced by the animal trembling or shaking, or by trying to record the ECG in a standing animal (Fig. 17.2). Purring in a cat (Fig. 17.3) will also result in baseline 'trembling'!

To correct this problem:

- Ensure the limbs are relaxed and supported.
- Find a position in which the animal will relax best, preferably not standing. Oftentimes a sitting position is good, and in some occasions, laying the animal on its side, with or without some manual restraint is required.
- Try holding the limbs to minimise the tremor.
- To stop a cat purring: dab a little spirit on the cat's nose using cotton wool.

Small Animal ECGs: An Introductory Guide, Third Edition. Mike Martin.
© 2015 John Wiley & Sons, Ltd. Published 2015 by John Wiley & Sons, Ltd.

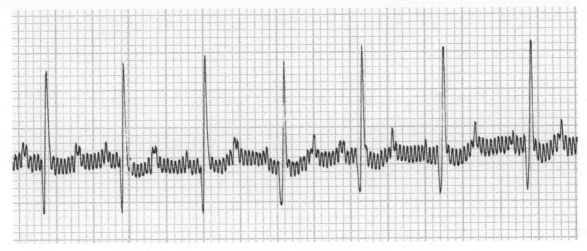

Figure 17.1 ECG showing 50-cycle alternating current interference artefact (which masks the P waves in this example).

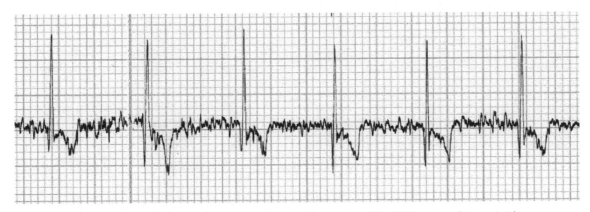

Figure 17.2 ECG showing muscle tremor artefact, which masks the P waves and makes interpretation difficult (25 mm/s and 10 mm/mV).

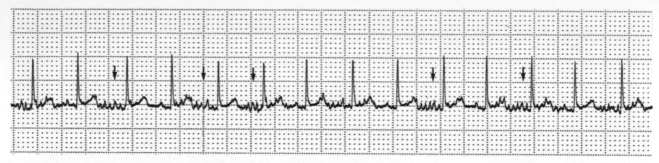

Figure 17.3 ECG from a cat with intermittent 'purring' artefact (25 mm/s and 10 mm/mV).

(a)

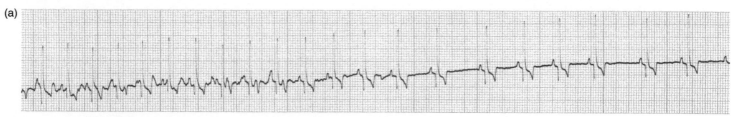

Figure 17.4 A selection of movement artefacts that make interpretation difficult (all tracings at 25mm/s and 1cm/mV, except in Fig. 17.4d). (a) ECG from a panting dog. Note the irregular movement of the baseline, then half way through the recording, the mouth of the dog is closed and the movement artefact stops; P waves are now recognisable.

(b)

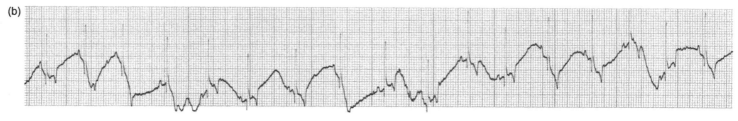

Figure 17.4 (b) ECG from a dog with dyspnoea associated with the foreleg ECG clips being attached too high up the leg and close to the chest. The chest movement causes movement of the forelimb clips and the up and down movement of the baseline.

(c)

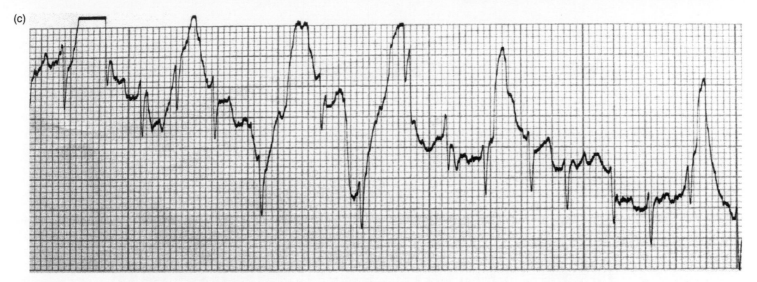

Figure 17.4 (c) ECG from a dog in which the ECG clip connection to the skin was loose and unstable, resulting in so much movement artefact that the tracing was non-diagnostic.

(d)

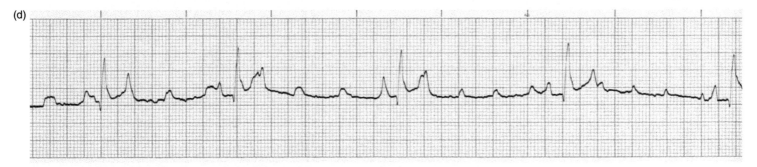

Figure 17.4 (d) ECG from a dog, in which the P-like movement artefacts create an effect that mimics heart block (50 mm/s and 10 mm/mV).

127

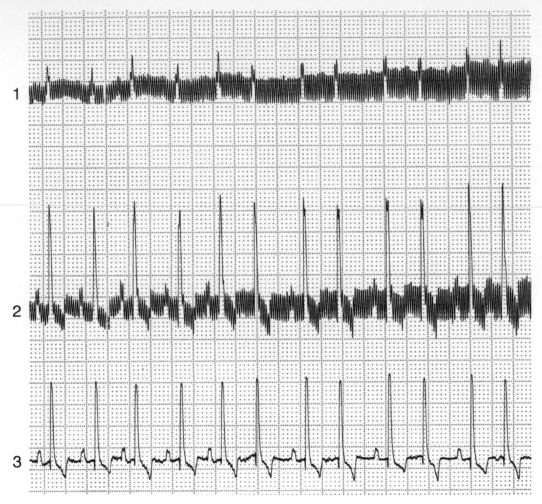

Figure 17.5 ECG from a dog with marked electrical interference in leads 1 and 2 (these tracings are unreadable), but lead 3 is of good quality. With the understanding of how the limb leads are created (see Fig. 9.1 in Chapter 9), it is possible to work out which electrode is inadequately connected to the skin. Leads 1 and 2 are common to the right fore – therefore, this is the electrode that needs attention (e.g. re-connecting or more spirit/gel applied). Alternatively, lead 3 is unaffected, and since that is created between the left fore and the left hind, these electrodes must have a good connection to the skin, leaving the right fore as the odd one out.

Movement artefact

This is a more exaggerated form of tremor artefact, but in this case, the deflections are not fine but variable and large. The stylus moves up and down the paper, which might be associated with respiratory movement (Fig. 17.4) or if the animal is moving or struggling.

To correct this problem:

- Correction of this is similar to tremor artefact.
- Try to get the animal to relax and remain still.
- Ensure the ECG cables are not moving with the movement of the animal, for example, respiratory movement (Chapter 18), or because the clips are not stable and secure.

Which leg moved?

With the aid of the diagrams in Chapter 9, it is possible to determine which leg is moving or causing connection problems. For example, if interference is seen in leads I and II, then the connection that is common to these leads is the right fore (Fig. 17.5). Therefore, this connection needs to be checked and the connection improved or the leg held still. If interference is seen in leads I and III, then the left fore needs to be checked. And if interference is seen in leads II and III then the left hind needs to be checked.

Incorrectly placed electrodes

This may result in inverted complexes or a bizarre mean electrical axis (Fig. 17.6).

> **Tip**
>
> P waves are nearly always positive in leads I, II and III. Double-check the position of the ECG cables, and use the colour code chart in Chapter 9, if necessary.

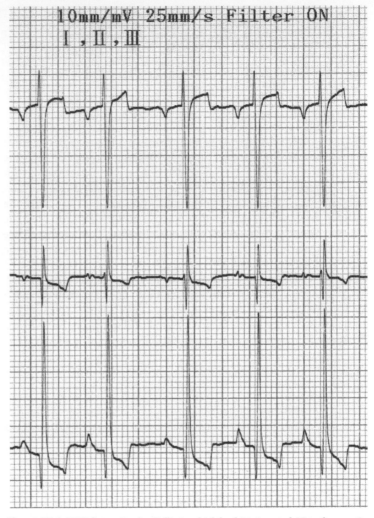

Figure 17.6 ECG from a Border Collie in which lead 1 is inverted. Note the negative P waves (as well as the negative QRS complexes). This was because the red and yellow forelimb electrodes where placed back to front.

18 • Recording an ECG

The connectors (electrodes)

To connect the ECG cable to the animal's skin requires a connector – this is called an **ECG electrode.** Since animals have a coat of hair, the commonly used human adhesive electrodes are not convenient for everyday regular use. Traditionally, the most commonly used electrodes to connect the ECG cable to the animal's skin has been the **crocodile clip**; however, while these provide good electrical connection, their bite can be painful to less stoical animals. There are now more suitable alternatives such as the **ECG Comfort Clip**, the **ECG Soft Clip** and the **ECG Vet Clip** (Fig. 18.1).

Human adhesive electrodes are routinely used for Holter recordings. A patch of hair is shaved, the skin is cleaned with spirit and then dried and the adhesive electrodes are applied. Adhesive electrodes can also be used on the paws of animals for longer-term monitoring during anaesthesia, for example (attached to the central pad and held in place with tape).

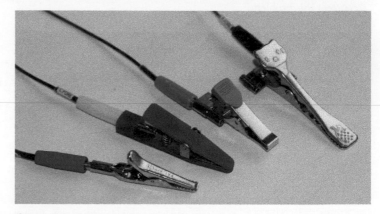

Figure 18.1 Photograph showing a selection of ECG clips currently available in the veterinary market. From left to right: the traditional crocodile clip, the Comfort clip, the Soft clip and the Vet clip.

Making the connection

This is the single most important part of ECG recording to obtain a good diagnostic quality tracing. The author routinely uses the ECG soft clip, so the following discussion will be based on this. But if you have decided to use an alternative electrode, then adapt the description accordingly.

Small Animal ECGs: An Introductory Guide, Third Edition. Mike Martin.
© 2015 John Wiley & Sons, Ltd. Published 2015 by John Wiley & Sons, Ltd.

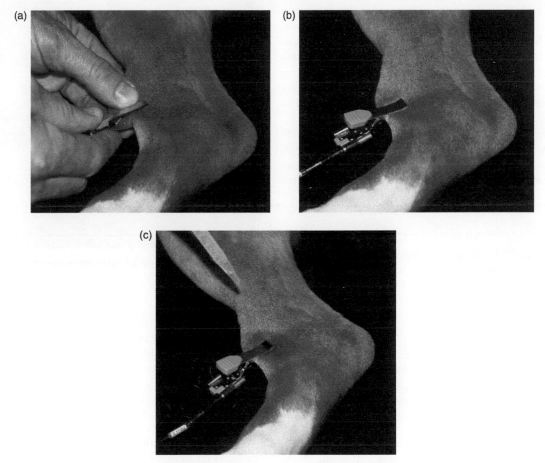

Figure 18.2 Placing an ECG clip to the skin of a dog (at the flexor angle of hock in this instance). Pinch a good piece of skin and position the ECG clip with its jaws fully open and over the skin as far as possible (a) such that the clips maintains a good bite of skin (b), and therefore, there is a good clip–skin contact. Spirit/alcohol can be applied to improve the contact between the clip and the skin through the hair/fur (c).

131

Using spirit

It is often sufficient with ECG clips to pick up a fold of skin between a finger and thumb (rolling the skin to feel its edge through a hairy coat) and with the other hand, open the ECG clip maximally, part the hair and attach the clip to the skin (Fig. 18.2). To obtain good conduction between the skin and the ECG clip requires the addition of a conducting medium – spirit is often adequate. Squirt a small amount of spirit (or alcohol), just sufficient to wet the ECG clip and through the hair to the skin.

However, spirit evaporates after 5–10 min, so this method would not suffice if the ECG recording takes longer than expected (such as during anaesthetic monitoring). Additionally, if spirit does not produce a good-quality, artefact-free recording, then an alternative method needs to be considered.

Using gel

Shave the site where the ECG clip is to be placed and attach the ECG clips. Then rub a gel on the clip and around it onto the skin (Fig. 18.3). Suitable gels are ECG gel, ultrasound gel or K-Y jelly.

Where to place the electrodes

In each animal, you need to pinch the skin at various sites on the limbs, preferably with least hair, to find a fold of loose skin. It is best to avoid the area where the skin is quite tight around the limb.

Forelegs

In the author's experience, the flexor angle of the elbow is a useful site (Fig. 18.4). An alternative site is caudal and just dorsal to the elbow.

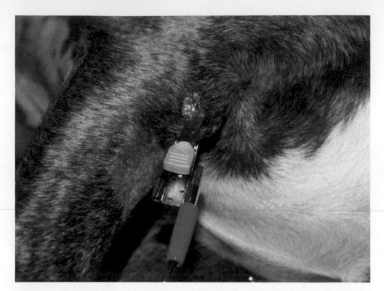

Figure 18.3 Alternatively, gel can be applied over the clip and around the skin after placement of the ECG clip.

However, since this is close to the chest, respiratory movement can result in movement of the cable and clip; thus, the ECG recording may be spoiled by movement artefact. Another site is halfway between the elbow and the carpus, on the palmar aspect of the leg.

Hind legs

In the author's experience, the flexor angle of the hock (or sometimes just above it) is a useful site (Fig. 18.4). Alternative sites are either above or below the knee, on the dorsal aspect of the limb.

How to position the ECG cables

In addition to the aforementioned, it is prudent not to place the ECG clips such that the cable runs over the animal, which can lead to respiratory movement artefact (as mentioned earlier) or to then twist the cable and ultimately the clip and the skin – even stoical animals may not tolerate this. When applying the ECG clip, have the ECG cable positioned away from the animal (Fig. 18.4) and resting on the table (or ground).

Positioning the animal

To minimise the electrical activity of the skeletal muscles, the animal must be relaxed and resting. If the animal trembles, shakes, pants or purrs, then all these activities will be manifest on the ECG, resulting in baseline artefact. This may hide small ECG complexes such as P waves or mimic the ECG activity. Thus, a good-quality ECG will have minimal movement, and there should be a steady baseline in between each ECG complex.

If the animal would be put at risk (e.g. if it was in respiratory distress) by making it adopt a position that it would not tolerate, then an ECG should be recorded in whatever position is achievable.

Dogs

Dogs are preferably placed in right lateral recumbency (Fig. 18.4). In many dogs, a recumbent position will reduce the skeletal muscle electrical activity and the 'normal values' for the dog ECG have been determined based on this position. If measurement of amplitudes are not critical, such as when examining primarily an arrhythmia, then recording an ECG while the dog lies, sits or even stands is acceptable, provided a good-quality tracing with minimal baseline movement artefact can be obtained.

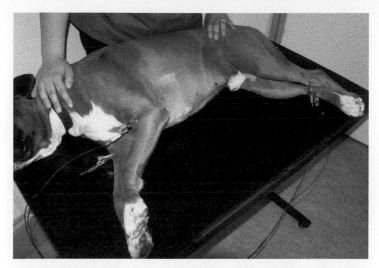

Figure 18.4 A Boxer dog having an ECG recording in right lateral recumbency using ECG clips, with the cables running away from the dog resting on an insulated table. A useful site of attachment for the ECG clips on the forelimbs is the skin at the flexor angle of the elbow and for the hind limbs is the skin at the flexor angle of the hock.

Isolating the electrodes

Once all the electrodes have been attached, it is essential to ensure that each ECG clip, the skin to which it is attached and the conducting medium (e.g. the spirit or gel), are not touching any other part of the animal, or the handler or the table (Fig. 18.4). This has the potential to cause electrical shorting and introduce artefacts into the ECG recording.

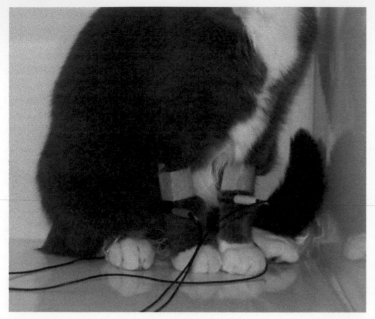

Figure 18.5 A cat having an ECG recording using paediatric limb electrodes, which have been held in place with tape. The inside of the metal can be soaked with spirit or gel.

Cats

The normal values for cats have not been determined in a lateral recumbent position; thus, recumbent positioning is less important. Many cats will often sit in a hunched position quite still (Fig. 18.5) – but each individual cat is different, and the veterinary surgeon must determine how each cat prefers to keep still. In fractious cats (and if the electrodes can be placed), putting the cat back in a basket together with the electrodes attached and ECG cables until it settles is a useful method. When, or if, the cat settles, the ECG can be recorded while the cat sits in the

basket. However, this method should, of course, be aborted if the cat starts to bite the ECG cables. Often, cats do resent the ECG clips, in which case, shaving a patch of hair and bandaging in place the adhesive electrodes or metal paediatric limb electrodes is easier, although it is more time consuming (Fig. 18.5).

> ### A word on Chemical restraint
>
> All sedative and tranquilliser drugs have a variable effect on the heart and/or autonomic tone. Drugs can, therefore, change the rate and rhythm of the heart directly or through effects on the autonomic tone. So, if you are performing an ECG to determine what the arrhythmia is that you heard, then there is a possibility that this will change if a chemical restraint is used. Ideally, therefore, any form of chemical restraint should be avoided when recording an ECG. If chemical restraint cannot be avoided then, based on physical examination, determine the rate and rhythm before and after using the drugs, and any differences should be taken into account when interpreting the ECG recording.

Setting up and preparing the ECG machine

This will vary slightly between different ECG machines, and adjustments to the following guidelines (which are based on a standard ECG machine) should be allowed.

Paper speed

Select the paper speed. Options are usually 25 and 50 mm/s. The paper speed selection is partly dependent on the animal's heart rate. As a guide: for normal heart rates in dogs, set the speed at 25 mm/s, but if there is a fast heart rate (and for cats), set the paper speed at 50 mm/s. In ECG machines with a computer-type print-out that produces a steppiness in

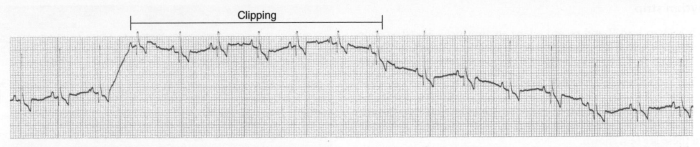

Figure 18.6 ECG showing the effect of clipping. Note the baseline drifts upwards (associated with movement) until the QRS complexes are restricted by the limits of the stylus; this is termed clipping (25 mm/s and 10 mm/mV).

the lines (i.e. pixel effect), measurement of ECG complex durations is best achieved at 100 mm/s.

Calibration

This is usually set at 1 cm/mV. However, if the complexes are very small, this can be increased to 2 cm/mV, and if the complexes are very large, it can be reduced to 0.5 cm/mV. In some machines, the calibration can be marked on the ECG paper by briefly running the ECG paper and pressing the 1 mV marker button – found on most standard ECG recorders.

Filter setting

Ideally, if good connections have been made, this can usually be left off, that is, without filter. Additionally, amplitude measurement should always be performed in an unfiltered tracing, as the dampening effect of the filter will reduce the amplitude of the complexes by a variable, although small, amount. If primarily examining for an arrhythmia and there is baseline artefact that cannot seem to be avoided, then filtering can reduce the baseline artefact and make reading of the ECG tracing easier.

Positioning the stylus

During the recording, the stylus should be positioned (if this is manually operated on the ECG machine) such that the whole of the ECG complex is within the 'graph lines' of the ECG paper. If the ECG produces particularly large complexes that run off the 'graph paper' (or outside the limits of the stylus or paper) this is referred to as **clipping** (Fig. 18.6). Remember then to move the stylus, up or down, such that the whole of the ECG tracing is within the graph paper (and not extending into the white margins) or alternatively reduce the calibration – whichever is more appropriate.

Recording an ECG – a suggested routine

10 seconds of all six limb leads

Run the ECG on each of the six bipolar leads, I, II, III, aVR, aVL and aVF, each for approximately 10 seconds. In order to ensure that each lead is well centred within the 'graph lines' of the ECG paper, briefly pause the ECG paper (with the stylus still moving) when switching the ECG machine from one lead to the next, until the stylus can be re-positioned as described earlier.

A rhythm strip

Switch back to lead II and record a long rhythm strip, 30–60 seconds, depending on each individual case requirement. If you have auscultated an occasional abnormal beat, then the ECG rhythm strip will need to be run until the abnormal beat is repeated. If lead II does not produce a good-quality tracing with satisfactorily large complexes, then run a rhythm strip on a lead that does. Or if you are searching for P waves (which can often be small and hard to see), then run the limb lead in which these are best shown.

A representative rhythm strip – this is really important!

If you auscultated what you thought was an arrhythmia, but it is not revealed on the ECG rhythm strip, then simultaneously auscultate the animal while continuing to run the ECG recording. It might be that the abnormality is only intermittently present, in which case you may have to continue to auscultate the animal until the arrhythmia is heard and hopefully captured on ECG. Maybe the arrhythmia is still audible on auscultation but not recognised on the ECG – in this case, the ECG tracing should be sent to a cardiologist for interpretation. Or, the abnormal heart sounds heard may not be an arrhythmia but, for example, could be a gallop sound. In summary, ensure that the ECG recording obtained is representative of what you found on physical examination.

Often, it is best to perform an ECG recording at the time of consultation, while the arrhythmia is present, because the arrhythmia can be intermittent and it only takes a couple of minutes (Fig. 18.7).

Label the tracing

Ensure the ECG recording is well labelled (unless the ECG machine does this automatically), either for future reference, or for other colleagues within your practice to be able to examine the recording, or in case you need to submit the tracing to a cardiologist for interpretation.

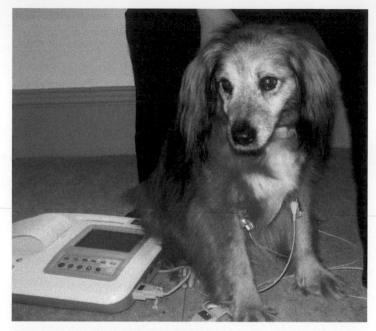

Figure 18.7 An ECG being performed during a consultation at the feet of the owner. Arrhythmias can be intermittent, and delaying the recording of an ECG might mean missing the opportunity to diagnose the arrhythmia.

Checklist

- State in which position the animal was restrained.
- Note paper speed and if, and where, it was changed.
- Note calibration and if, and where, it was changed.
- Label filter level, and when, and where, it was used.
- Label each lead at its beginning.
- State if any chemical restraint was used.

19 • Choosing an ECG recorder

In attempting to put down on paper some advice on choosing an ECG recorder – which is a question often asked of the author – I can only describe my own personal preferences and opinions. Other cardiologists may have different viewpoints and opinions.

An ECG machine required for diagnostic purposes is preferably a recorder that prints onto paper rather than a monitor that is viewed on a screen or computer. In other words, using an ECG monitor (used in perianaesthetic or intensive care monitoring) is not ideal for diagnostic ECG recordings. It is best to have a separate recorder for diagnostic electrocardiography and a monitor for anaesthesia.

Quality

This is the most important factor. Recorders should produce a good-quality high-resolution tracing such that no pixelation (stepping) is evident. Older computerised recordings tended to produce a pixelated print-out (Fig. 19.1a) and occasionally ECG recorders that print onto ECG tracing paper, yet the print-out is pixelated (Fig. 19.1b). Any pixelation in the tracing will affect the ability to recognise important small deflections, in particular when searching for P waves.

Continuous recording

The ability to record a continuous paper trace without interruption and in real time is preferred. This is not possible, for example, with machines and computers that print out onto sheets of A4 paper. This will mean an ECG recorder with either paper in rolls or Z-fold paper. However, sometimes Z-fold paper can fail to adequately allow scribing of a deflection on the fold itself (Fig. 19.2), although this paper is easy for storing, compared with paper rolls.

Small Animal ECGs: An Introductory Guide, Third Edition. Mike Martin.
© 2015 John Wiley & Sons, Ltd. Published 2015 by John Wiley & Sons, Ltd.

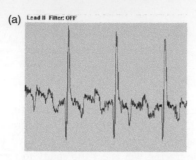

(a) Lead II Filter: OFF

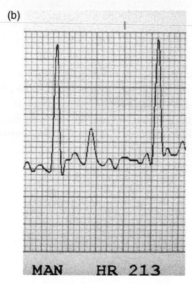

(b)

I

MAN   **HR 213**

Figure 19.1 (a) A low-resolution computer tracing in which the combination of pixilation and movement artefact makes interpretation impossible. (b) A low-resolution computerised print-out onto ECG paper, again with pixilation making interpretation difficult. These types of machines are best avoided.

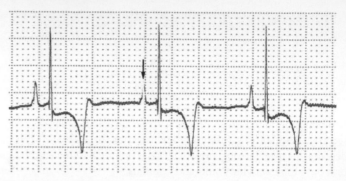

Figure 19.2 ECG showing a sinus rhythm of three complexes; however, the P wave of the middle complex (arrowed) is partly hidden on the fold of the z-fold paper.

Ease of use

The recorder is simple and intuitive to use, that is, not so complex that a detailed users' manual is required to understand it.

Automatic labelling

It is very useful to purchase a machine that performs automatic labelling, on the paper, showing the calibration, paper speed and filter level (Fig. 19.3). It is also best if any alteration to the settings is labelled immediately following a change rather than at fixed intervals.

Automatic versus manual recording mode

My preference is to work in manual mode, with the ability to change the leads when appropriate. Automatic mode means that the recorder runs through each of the leads, recording a set duration, often short, for each lead. If automatic mode is used, it is useful to know how to stop the recording before attempting to print out unattached *precordial chest*

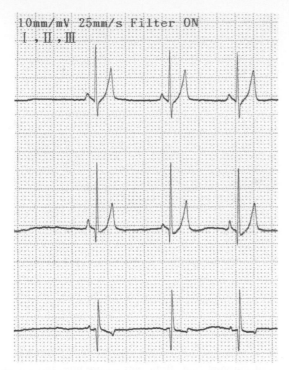

10mm/mV 25mm/s Filter ON
I , II , III

Figure 19.3 Automatic labelling of the lead, paper speed and calibration is a useful feature. In this three-channel recorder, the calibration (10 mm/mV), speed (25 mm/s), filter level (on) and ECG leads (1, 2 and 3) are automatically printed.

leads, or when the dog moves, or how to perform a continuous lead II rhythm strip.

Interpretative software

This does not appear to work reliably in animals: primarily due to attempts at interpreting baseline artefacts, particularly movement artefact. I have seen a number of owners referred on the basis of misleading or wrong computer interpretation, such that I would be of the opinion that this should be avoided, except in the hands of someone experienced (in which case, interpretation is not required!).

Multichannel versus single channel

Multichannel recorders permit the simultaneous recording of more than one lead at a time, most commonly three leads, for example, leads I, II and III. If a leg moves during a recording, sometimes, this can mimic an ectopic (Fig. 19.4), but in a three-channel recording, usually one lead will remain unaffected and thus reveal that the cardiac rhythm was normal.

Paper width

Paper width is important when opting for a multichannel recorder. Some machines print out three (and sometimes four) leads on fairly miserly paper width, resulting in the top and bottoms of QRS complexes overlapping (Fig. 19.5a). This can make interpretation challenging. Halving the sensitivity is less than an ideal way to get round this problem on a regular basis. So if choosing a multichannel recorder, choose one with respectably wide paper, which I would suggest should be >10 cm.

It is also preferable that the machine is set up such that there is not a repeat of the lead II as a rhythm strip, creating a fourth channel and further compromising on space (Fig. 19.5b).

Precordial chest leads

These are generally not required for animal use. I occasionally use a single precordial lead in search of small deflections, such as P waves. But this is rarely required, and the additional leads create an added storage problem.

139

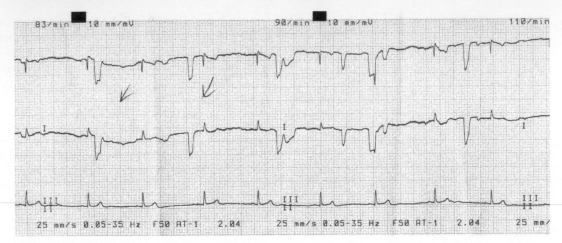

Figure 19.4 A multichannel recorder helps identify movement artefact that might mimic an ectopic. In this example from a cat, the vet has arrowed deflections for a second opinion that look like ventricular ectopics. However, these only affect leads 1 and 2, but not lead 3. These are, therefore, artefacts as a result of movement affecting the ECG clip to right foreleg.

Calibration settings

The standard paper speed settings are 25 and 50 mm/s. Other speeds (5, 12.5 or 100 mm/s) are sometimes additionally available – these can occasionally be useful options, but are not essential.

The standard amplitude sensitivity is 10 mm/mV. A double sensitivity of 20 mm/mV is useful when the complexes are quite small, such as with cats. A half sensitivity of 5 mm/mV is required when the QRS complexes are very tall in some dogs that might have cardiomegaly.

A filter is often required in animals to reduce the baseline artefact noise from electrical interference of muscle tremor. One filter level is usually sufficient, although some machines provide two filter levels.

Automatic centring versus manual control

Control of the stylus can be performed either manually (usually in older recorders) or automatically. Both options are fine, and the automatic centring in new machines usually works well, despite animal movement.

Internal battery

This is a useful feature and, in most machines, comes as standard, which means you can take the ECG machine to a patient without worry about finding a nearby electrical socket

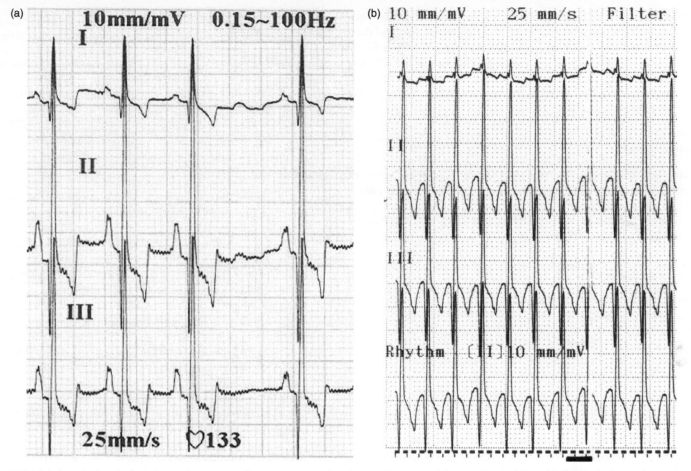

(a)

10mm/mV 0.15~100Hz

I

II

III

25mm/s ♡133

(b) 10 mm/mV   25 mm/s   Filter

I

II

III

Rhythm [II] 10 mm/mV

Figure 19.5 (a) A three-lead multichannel recorder on 7 cm tall paper; it is just a bit of a miserly squeeze and can make rhythm analysis difficult, due to the overlap of the deflections. (b) ECG from a dog, again with the ECG complexes overlapping each other, making interpretation difficult. In this case, lead 2 is repeated on the fourth line, which is unnecessary and if turned off, there would be more room for the standard three limb leads (1, 2 and 3).

Jack plug lead fitting

The most common method to connect to the skin of dogs has been crocodile clips. However, these can be painful to some animals, and there are now a wide range of effective but gentler options. These include: the Comfy Clip, Soft Clip, Vet Clips, paediatric limb plates and adhesive electrodes (Fig. 18.6). The press stud fittings are of limited use in animals; in humans they are used for attaching to circular adhesive electrodes, but adaptors for these are also available now.

Monitor screen

This is a very useful option. It means the ECG rhythm can be monitored for long periods without printing to paper (and thus wasting paper). Machines that have a memory function are useful in this setting, because an arrhythmia seen on the screen can then be printed out for the record or posted for an expert interpretation.

Thermal paper versus ink paper

Thermal sensitive paper is more practical compared to ink paper, avoiding the need for replacement ink at difficult or busy times. Thermal paper that turns black (rather than blue) usually provides better contrast for scanning. However, some papers do not have a long-term retention (>1 year) of the image recorded, which gradually fades over time – something to watch for and try to avoid.

New versus second-hand

While a new ECG recorder is the ideal, the cost of this can prevent some practices from purchasing an ECG machine – which would be 'the greater of two evils'! If cost is a limiting factor, then a second-hand machine can be a good option. In these cases, it is important to have the machine serviced prior to use. If the machine comes without leads, there are companies that can make these up.

> **Tip**
>
> Sometimes it is useful to create an electronic copy of an ECG paper tracing, either for your own record, or for publication in a book or article, or to submit by email to a colleague for a second opinion. An effective method is to use a flatbed colour scanner, set in photo-mode, scanning at 600dpi (pixels per inch). The file can be saved in jpeg format and suitably cropped and labelled with standard image software.

My ideal veterinary ECG machine would have the following features

- A three-channel recording machine, able to switch between lead 1, 2 and 3, or between aVR, aVL and aVF, or a precordial chest lead (run as a fourth channel).
- A monitor screen in which the sweep speed is not too fast, 25mm/s is usually sufficient.
- Memory recording over a 30 second loop, so that the screen can be viewed until an arrhythmia occurs and then printed.
- Paper width of >10 cm.
- A high resolution tracing with no pixelation.
- Continuous real-time recording.
- Calibration settings: pre-set to 25 mm/s, 10mm/mV and filter off.
- Ease of use and intuitive to use with the facility to change the leads, paper speed, calibration and filter, with one-touch buttons (without going into a menu system).
- Automatic labelling of the leads, paper speed, calibration and filter level at the start, regular intervals and following any change.
- The machine to work in 'manual' mode.
- Internal battery (can run off-mains).
- Jack plug fittings to the ends of the electrodes, with suitable ECG clips.
- The ability to store the ECG recording digitally on a computer.
- No interpretive software.

20 • Ambulatory ECG monitoring

A routine in-clinic ECG is recorded for a relatively short period of time, usually less than 5 minutes. However, some intermittent arrhythmias, suspected to be the cause of clinical signs such as collapse, may not occur during a 5 minutes ECG recording. In these cases, then a much longer ECG recording is required to capture the arrhythmia leading to a collapse. A Holter recorder would be the most common method of recording these long periods. Additionally, small sterile loop recorders can be implanted under the skin to monitor the ECG during an 'event' such as collapse. This chapter addresses the useful and practical aspects of these ECG devices.

Holter monitors

A Holter is a small, portable, battery-operated recorder, which stores the ECG on a memory card (Fig. 20.1). It can continuously record an ECG for as little as an hour up to several days (depending upon the capacity of the memory card) but most commonly for 24 hours. The patient can carry on normal day-to-day activities while at home or re-enact situations that have triggered collapses. The use of more than one lead allows for the differentiation of artefact (which is unlikely to appear

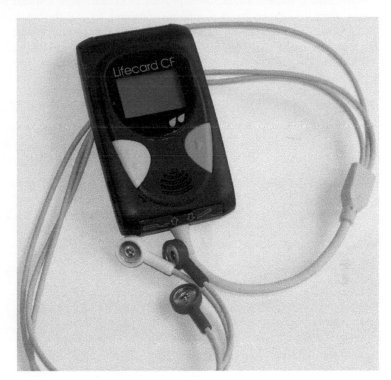

Figure 20.1 Photograph of a commonly used Holter monitor in veterinary cardiology practice.

Small Animal ECGs: An Introductory Guide, Third Edition. Mike Martin.
© 2015 John Wiley & Sons, Ltd. Published 2015 by John Wiley & Sons, Ltd.

in all leads) and also increases the likelihood of a good recording (as occasionally, one of the leads may be non-diagnostic).

The recording is reviewed on a computer using the manufacturer's software. Automated full disclosure software is available; however, it is expensive and requires an experienced operator, and thus many will use a company providing an interpretation and analysis service (that also hires monitors out). Some manufacturers provide ECG disclosure software (often much less expensive than analysis software), so that the whole ECG recording can be viewed on a computer (but does not provide a quantitative analysis). This can be particularly useful if looking for 'events' such as collapse and if the time of the event is known from the owner's diary. Additionally, some Holter recorders have an 'event' button on the device, which can be activated by the owner when their pet collapses and is marked on the recording – this is particularly useful and highly recommended.

Indications for Holter monitoring

Collapse, syncope, pre-syncope and episodic weakness

Holter monitoring enables the detection of intermittent arrhythmias and so might reveal the cause of events such as syncope or episodic weakness.

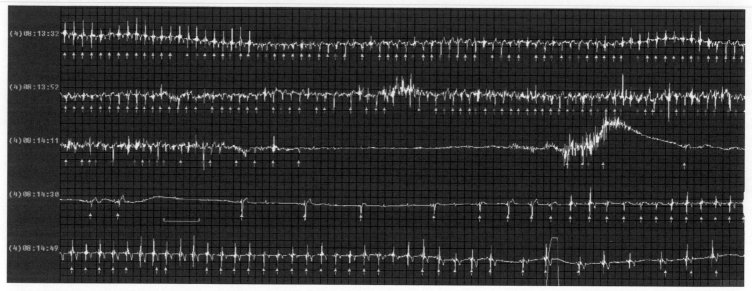

Figure 20.2 Holter recording from a Whippet that had a history of collapse, which was unclear whether it was a cardiac syncope or seizure. During the collapse, the owner presses the 'event marker' button (green mark on line 4); preceding this, it can be seen that there is a period of sinus arrest causing the collapse. Movement artefact is noted towards the end of the third line of tracing as the dog collapses.

It is most effective when an event occurs while the Holter is worn. The time of the event must be accurate and recorded either by using the 'event button' on the Holter (Fig. 20.2) or noting the time. When the patient does not have an event during the recording, arrhythmias may be detected that provide a clue as to the likely cause of the collapse. However, if there were no arrhythmias during the recording, then repeated Holter monitoring, or the use of an implantable loop recorder, may be required.

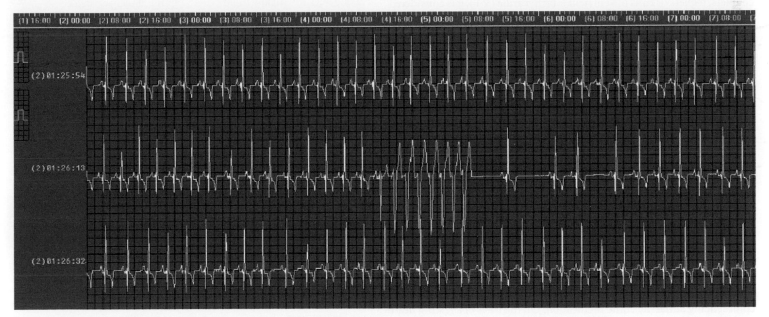

Figure 20.3 Holter recording from a Doberman showing paroxysmal ventricular tachycardia that was not seen on an in-clinic resting ECG.

Screening ventricular arrhythmias

Holter monitoring is indicated for detecting ventricular arrhythmias in dogs suspected of having cardiomyopathy or breed screening schemes, particularly in predisposed breeds such as Boxers and Dobermans (Figs 20.3 & 20.4). Patients with degenerative mitral valve disease have also been shown to experience increasing arrhythmia with severity of disease. In this situation, the Holter monitor is worn for 24 hours and the number of ventricular arrhythmias per 24 hours counted. Less than 50 VPCs per 24 hours is often considered within normal limits. A simplified guideline on the classification of the number of arrhythmias or complexity is provided in the following table (Table 20.1).

In Dobermans > 50 VPCs per 24 h, particularly if there are also couplets, triplets or runs of ventricular tachycardia (VT), it is considered likely to be associated with cardiomyopathy.

In Boxer dogs, ARVC is associated with ventricular arrhythmias and criteria have been suggested (Table 20.2).

Monitoring therapy for tachyarrhythmias

A Holter is recorded prior to and then 1–2 weeks after commencing antiarrhythmic medication for both ventricular and supraventricular arrhythmias. A good response is considered to be a reduction in the number of VPCs by >80% and a significant reduction in episodes of VT with a significant clinical response.

Monitoring therapy for atrial fibrillation

One of the criteria for treatment of atrial fibrillation is to reduce the heart rate response, which is conventionally considered to be <160/min. However, the in-clinic heart rate is significantly more than the rate measured at home. One of the more reliable ways to determine the heart rate is therefore a 24 hour Holter, performed before and then 1 week after commencing antiarrhythmic medication. On the basis of a resting heart rate at home, a reasonable heart rate response is likely to be <120/min.

Table 20.1   Simplified guidelines on the classification[1] of ventricular arrhythmias on Holter monitoring, when considering antiarrhythmic therapy. This can be based on a combination of the number of VPCs per 24 h and/or the complexity of the ventricular arrhythmia. Animals with 'severe' complexity are generally considered to be the ones at greatest risk of sudden death.

Severity	Number of VPCs per 24 h	Complexity
Normal	<50	Single VPCs, mostly monomorphic.
Mild	50–1000	Pairs and triplets, non-sustained runs of VT, mostly monomorphic.
Moderate	1000–10,000	The above + sustained runs of VT, often polymorphic.
Severe	>10,000	The above + Sustained runs of very fast VT often with R-on-T, polymorphic VPCs or VT

[1] There are no specific publications or agreement to define severity; this is a simplified guideline based on the author's experience, with the aim of providing some guidance to the practitioner.

Table 20.2   Criteria for Holter monitor screening of Boxer dogs.

VPCs per 24 h	Interpretation
0–50	Normal
51–100	Indeterminate
100–300	Suspicious
100–300 + couplets, triplets and VT	Likely affected
300–1000	Likely affected
> 1000	Affected

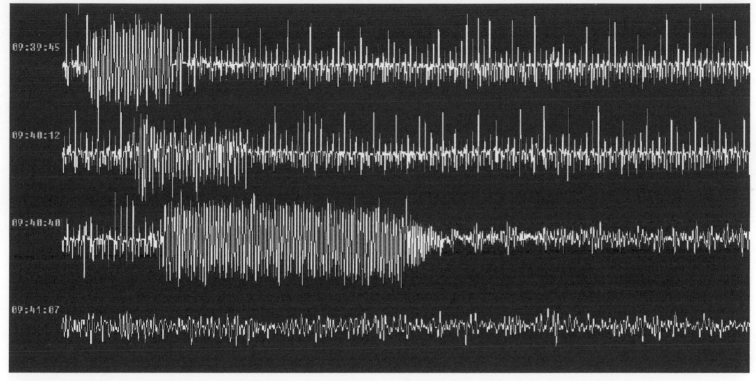

Figure 20.4 Holter from a Doberman that has very fast episodes of ventricular tachycardia (lines 1 and 2) in between periods of sinus rhythm and then a longer period of ventricular tachycardia (line 3) that degenerated into ventricular fibrillation, resulting in sudden death.

How to fit a Holter monitor on animals

- The hair over the sites for placement of the electrodes needs to be clipped and degreased with surgical spirit and then dried.
- The +ve electrode is placed over the left apex, another low on the right thorax and the third high on either the right or left thorax (Fig. 20.5).

- Adhesive electrodes are stuck to the skin and the leads from the Holter attached.
- The leads (and Holter) can be held in place by adhesive bandaging (Fig. 20.6a) or a commercially available Holter vest (Fig. 20.6b).
- When using bandages, it is useful to place the monitor in a plastic bag to protect it from the adhesive and moisture and also create a

(a) (b)

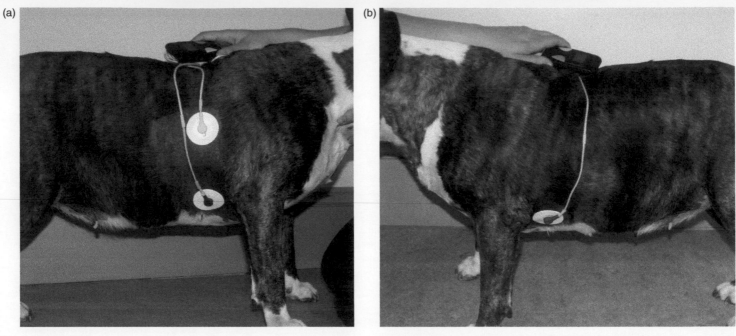

Figure 20.5 (a, b) Photographs of an English Bull Terrier being fitted with a Holter monitor. In this instance, two electrodes are attached to the right thorax and one to the left (over the apex beat).

window such that the screen and buttons can be seen. The bandages can be removed with the aid of an adhesive solvent such as Leukotape® Remover.
- If using a Holter vest, the monitor and leads need to be fed through the gaps in the vest and placed in the appropriate pouch, through which the owner can easily access the 'patient event' button on the monitor.
- It is important that the owner keeps a diary of the dog's periods of activity and rest, as well as any other events. Encourage them to

press the 'event button', record the time and describe the event on the diary.

Artefacts on Holter recordings

To the inexperienced eye, artefacts on Holter recordings can mimic arrhythmias. A dog scratching its chest when a Holter is strapped on can produce movement artefact that mimics a short burst of VT,

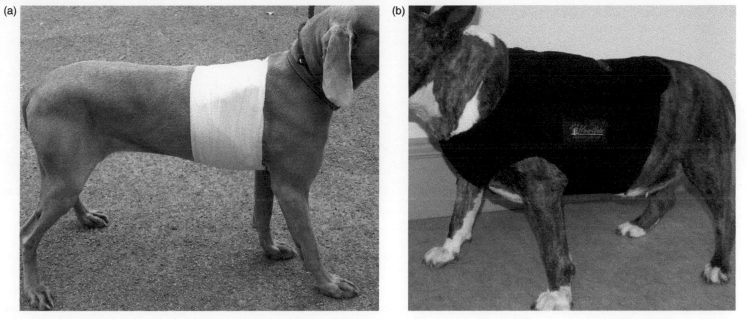

Figure 20.6 (a) Photograph of a Holter strapped on using adhesive bandaging, which provides secure and stable contact between the electrodes and the skin. The bandages can be removed with the aid of an adhesive solvent such as Leukotape remover. (b) Photograph of an English Bull Terrier fitted with a Holter monitor held in place by a commercially available vest.

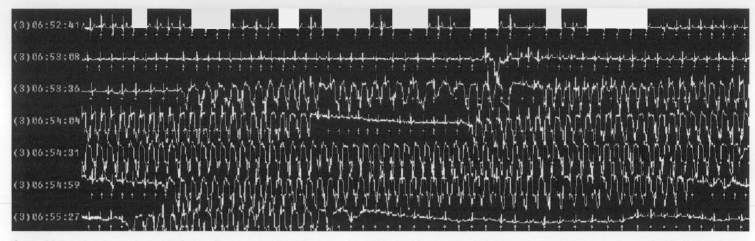

Figure 20.7 Holter from a dog in which the adhesive electrodes did not have adequate or stable contact with the skin. This resulted in a panting-artefact during exercise that mimicked periods of ventricular tachycardia.

or a loosely attached electrode can be affected by excessive breathing or panting, resulting in movement artefact (Fig. 20.7). Artefacts can also occur when an electrode loses a firm attachment or comes off, resulting in intermittent or no ECG recording. There is typically a lot of variation in the QRS amplitude as the dog lies in various positions throughout the day, but this is all considered normal. There is an extremely wide heart rate range considered normal in dogs, with rates between 30 and 300/min reported as normal, depending on the activity and physiologic state. Hence, experienced analysts are better placed to differentiate between normal and abnormal rhythms. Bradyarrhythmias such as exaggerated sinus arrhythmia, sinus pause (up to 7 seconds) and second-degree AVB are relatively common in dogs due to high resting vagal tone. Low numbers of SVPCs and VPCs occurring singly are also relatively considered normal.

Implantable loop recorder

An implantable loop recorder (ILR), such as the Medtronic Reveal, is a very small, sterile device that can be implanted under the skin near the heart (Fig. 20.8); the battery life is approximately 3 years. It is most usefully employed for cases in which there are infrequent episodes of collapse that have not been recorded on a 5–7 day Holter.

A programmer is required to preset the ECG storage options within the device. The ILP can be set to store a number of 'patient activated recordings', which is the most useful feature in animals. It can also be programmed to automatically store ECG recordings based on human upper and lower heart rate limits, but these are often not sufficient for the greater range of rates seen in animals.

The ILR continuously records a single lead ECG but following an event, the owner uses a handheld device to activate storage of the ECG recording. The recorded loop is typically several minutes in duration and should capture the period of time leading up to and during a collapse.

Reading of the ECG recordings requires interpretation by the manufacturer's analyser device either by upload via the internet or directly with a programmer.

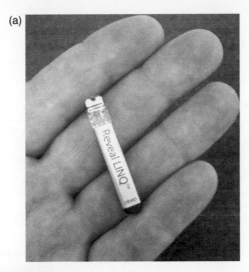

(a)

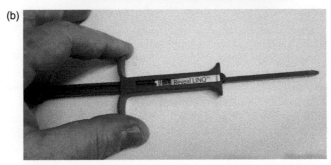

(b)

Figure 20.8 (a) Photograph of an implantable loop recorder (Medtronic Reveal LINQ). (b) Photograph shows the delivery device used for placement through a small incision in the skin.

Further reading

As a general reference guide, the following textbook is recommended:

L. P. Tilley (1992) *Essentials of Canine and Feline Electrocardiography: Interpretation and Treatment*, 3rd edn, Lea & Febiger.

For practising reading ECGs, the following books are strongly recommended:

L. P. Tilly and F. Smith (1993) *Canine and Feline Cardiac Arrythmias: Self Assessment*, Lippincott, Williams & Wilkins.

M. A. Oyama, M. S. Kraus and A. R. Gelzer (2014) *Rapid Review of ECG Interpretation in Small Animal Practice*, Taylor and Francis Group.

T. Day (2005) *ECG Interpretation in the Critically Ill Dog and Cat*, Blackwell Publishing.

An audiotape or CD:

F. W. K. Smith, B. W. Keane and L. P. Tilley (2005) *Rapid Interpretation of Heart and Lung Sounds: A Guide to Cardiac and Respiratory Auscultation in Dogs and Cats*, 2nd edn, Saunders.

C. Kvart and J. Haggstrom (2002) *Cardiac Auscultation and Phonocardiography in Dogs, Horses and Cats*, Clarence Kvart, Uppsala, Sweden.

Books on veterinary cardiology:

E. Cote, K. A. MacDonald, K. M. Meurs and M. M. Sleeper (2011) *Feline Cardiology*, Wiley-Blackwell.

P. Darke, J. D. Bonagura and D. F. Kelly (1996) *Color Atlas of Veterinary Cardiology*, Mosby-Wolfe.

P. R. Fox, D. Sisson and N. S. Moise (1999) *Textbook of Canine and Feline Cardiology*, 2nd edn, WB Saunders.

M. D. Kittleson and R. D. Kienle (1998) *Small Animal Cardiovascular Medicine*, Mosby.

V. Luis-Fuentes and S. Swift (1998) *Manual of Small Animal Cardiorespiratory Medicine and Surgery*, BSAVA, Cheltenham.

O. L. Nelson (2003) *Small Animal Cardiology*, Butterworth-Heinemann.

M. W. S. Martin and B. Corcoran (2006) *Notes on Cardiorespiratory Disease of the Dog and Cat*, 2nd edn, Blackwell Publishing.

L. P. Tilly, F. W. K. Smith, M. Oyama and M. M. Sleeper (2008) *Manual of Canine and Feline Cardiology*, 4th edn, Saunders.

O. L. Nelson (2001) *Small Animal Cardiology (The Practical Veterinarian)*, Butterworth-Heinemann Ltd.

B. W. Keane and R. Hamlin (1997) *Small Animal Cardiology*, Saunders.

W. A. Ware (2011) *Cardiovascular Disease in Small Animal Medicine*, 3rd edn, Manson Publishing.

Index

Small Animal ECGs: An Introductory Guide, Third Edition. Mike Martin.
© 2015 John Wiley & Sons, Ltd. Published 2015 by John Wiley & Sons, Ltd.